EMERGENCY NURSING

5-Tier Triage Protocols

Julie K. Briggs, BSN, RN, MHA, is a registered nurse with 40 years of experience in emergency nursing. She has provided nursing leadership in multiple hospital departments including emergency care, critical care, cardiac catheterization laboratory, radiology, and ambulatory care. Additional areas of expertise include disaster response, management and training, telephone triage training, program development, and consulting. Publications include *Emergency Nursing: 5-Tier Triage Protocols, Telephone Triage Protocols for Nurses,* editions 1–5, *Telephone Triage Protocols for Pediatrics,* and *Triage Protocols for Aging Adults.* In addition, Ms. Briggs has contributed multiple articles and book chapters in emergency nursing, leadership, and home health. She currently works at Providence Health Plan in Quality Management in Portland, Oregon.

Valerie Aarne Grossman, MALS, BSN, RN, NE-BC, is a registered nurse with four decades of heterogeneous nursing experience including bedside nursing, nursing leadership, and hospital administration. She is a nurse author and serves with multiple nursing organizations. Her areas of expertise include emergency nursing, telephone triage, radiology nursing, and nursing leadership. Ms. Aarne Grossman currently serves as the Vice-Chairperson for the New York State Board of Nursing (2019–2020) and the Chairperson (2020–2021). She volunteers for a number of organizations and boards of directors including the New York State Board of Nursing, the Association for Radiologic & Imaging Nursing (ARIN), and the *Journal of Radiology Nursing.* She is a prolific author of numerous books, chapters, and articles. She is a manuscript reviewer for journals from around the world. She is an award-winning nurse, most recently was named the ARIN Radiology Nurse of the Year, and received the American Nurses Association Honorary Nursing Practice Award. Her advocacy for the bedside nurse drives her passion for professional involvement and dedication to providing the profession of nursing with written tools that can help nurses reach their full potential in providing patient care.

SECOND EDITION

EMERGENCY NURSING

5-Tier Triage Protocols

Julie K. Briggs, BSN, RN, MHA

Valerie Aarne Grossman, MALS, BSN, RN, NE-BC

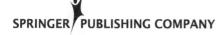
SPRINGER PUBLISHING COMPANY

Springer Publishing Company, LLC
11 West 42nd Street
New York, NY 10036
www.springerpub.com
http://connect.springerpub.com

Acquisitions Editor: Elizabeth Nieginski
Compositor: S4Carlisle Publishing Services

ISBN: 978-0-8261-3788-3
ebook ISBN: 978-0-8261-3791-3
DOI: 10.1891/9780826137913

Printed by BnT

The author and the publisher of this Work have made every effort to use sources believed to be reliable to provide information that is accurate and compatible with the standards generally accepted at the time of publication. Because medical science is continually advancing, our knowledge base continues to expand. Therefore, as new information becomes available, changes in procedures become necessary. We recommend that the reader always consult current research and specific institutional policies before performing any clinical procedure. The author and publisher shall not be liable for any special, consequential, or exemplary damages resulting, in whole or in part, from the readers' use of, or reliance on, the information contained in this book. The publisher has no responsibility for the persistence or accuracy of URLs for external or third-party Internet websites referred to in this publication and does not guarantee that any content on such websites is, or will remain, accurate or appropriate.

Library of Congress Cataloging-in-Publication Data

Names: Briggs, Julie K., author. | Grossman, Valerie G. A., author.
Title: Emergency nursing : 5-tier triage protocols / Julie K. Briggs,
    Valerie Aarne Grossman.
Description: Second edition. | New York : Springer Publishing Company,
    [2020] | Includes bibliographical references and index.
Identifiers: LCCN 2019029276 (print) | ISBN 9780826137883 (hardcover) |
    ISBN 9780826137913 (ebook)
Subjects: MESH: Emergency Nursing | Triage--methods | Emergencies--nursing
    | Emergency Service, Hospital | Handbook
Classification: LCC RC86.7 (print) | LCC RC86.7 (ebook) | NLM WY 49 |
    DDC 616.02/5--dc23
LC record available at https://lccn.loc.gov/2019029276
LC ebook record available at https://lccn.loc.gov/2019029277

Contact us to receive discount rates on bulk purchases.
We can also customize our books to meet your needs.
For more information please contact: sales@springerpub.com

Julie K. Briggs: https://orcid.org/0000-0001-7731-9819
Valerie Aarne Grossman: https://orcid.org/0000-0002-7648-7113

Printed in the United States of America.

CONTENTS

Protocols

Appendices

PREFACE

The process of triage occurs in a variety of settings around the world, from the battlefield to the private medical office. Each venue may have different goals and practices that are dependent on the location of the incident or place of service, patient care needs, and available medical resources. A triage process is essential to assist the care provider in prioritizing the needs of those seeking care, working to minimize or prevent a delay in care to the patient with the highest acuity risk. Triage methods and sources have evolved over many decades and now address the needs of different practice settings.

The Need for 5-Level Triage Protocols

Today, most healthcare organizations (emergency departments, urgent care centers, infirmaries, clinics, etc.) in countries around the world use some type of triage acuity system to determine how quickly a patient needs to be seen and who can safely wait until services are available to provide the necessary care. Over the past 10 to 15 years, many organizations have transitioned to a 5-Tier Acuity System. Some countries have developed their own triage system that consists of 3 to 5 levels of acuity. Do a quick Internet search and you will find a wide variety available—some are electronic and some continue to use pen and paper. In *Emergency Nursing: 5-Tier Triage Protocols* (Second Edition), the term "emergency department" is frequently used; however, all providers of healthcare that use a triage system will benefit from this valuable resource.

In today's rapidly changing healthcare environment, an efficient emergency department is critical to providing appropriate care at the appropriate time in the appropriate setting. A 5-level triage system helps to ensure that patients are not overtriaged, which depletes scarce resources that may be needed for a patient requiring immediate intervention, or undertriaged, which puts the patient at risk for deterioration while waiting to be seen.

Emergency Nursing: 5-Tier Triage Protocols will assist the triage nurse to function in a more consistent, reliable, and safe manner. The five levels are Resuscitation, Emergent, Urgent, Semi-urgent, and Nonurgent, and they are based on patient acuity, severity of symptoms, the degree of risk for deterioration while waiting, and the need for additional resources. In the protocols, ascending levels of urgency are indicated by bolder headings and shading.

This protocol manual can help to achieve the following goals:

- Provide consistency in triage decisions among different nurses
- Utilize healthcare resources in the most appropriate manner
- Set minimum expectations for triage decisions

- Guide the nurse in asking the right questions
- Assist the nurse in determining how soon the patient needs to be seen
- Remind the nurse of interventions to consider
- Serve as a reference for experienced nurses
- Aid the less experienced nurse in conducting the triage assessment
- Serve as a training tool in orientation
- Provide guidelines for designing and implementing a formal triage program
- Provide guidelines and tools for measuring and ensuring quality
- Provide additional information to expand the nurse's knowledge of key conditions, causes, and presentation to assist in the triage process
- Provide guidelines for the role of triage in disasters, multiple casualty incidents, and active shooter incidents

Protocol Components

Each protocol has been developed to ensure accuracy and consistency among the different protocols. Each protocol includes the following:

Title: Protocols are arranged alphabetically and are symptom-based. There are a few diagnosis-based protocols, such as diabetic problems or asthma, that are based on a known diagnosis or history.

Key Questions: These questions prompt the nurse to routinely ask for baseline and background information, to assist the nurse in providing the safest and most comprehensive assessment possible. Key Questions offer additional conditions and other influential factors, such as exposures, prior history, and prior treatment, to be considered when triaging each patient. It is always important to follow the policies of your facility, your scope of practice under your licensure, and all regulatory agency requirements. Other Key Questions are protocol-specific and prompt the nurse to measure oxygen saturation or ask about the mechanism of injury.

Acuity Level/Assessment and Nursing Considerations: The assessment is categorized from Level 1 through Level 5, with the most severe and life-threatening symptoms listed first in Level 1.

Level 1—Resuscitation: This category is critical and the patient's condition is life-threatening if not managed immediately. In assigning this acuity, the nurse should consider that the patient's condition could quickly deteriorate and will require multiple staff at the bedside, mobilization of the resuscitation team, and many resources. For providers that are not within a hospital, this will require a prompt call for emergency services to assist.

Level 2—Emergent: This category is high risk for a patient waiting for treatment. The patient's condition could deteriorate rapidly if treatment is delayed. In assigning this acuity, the nurse should consider that the patient will require multiple diagnostic studies or procedures, frequent consultation with the physician, and continuous monitoring. For providers that are not within a hospital, this will require a prompt call for emergency services to assist.

Level 3—Urgent: This category is moderate risk for a patient waiting to be seen. The patient's condition is stable, but treatment should be provided as soon as possible to relieve distress and pain. Each facility should determine acceptable waiting times if a room is not immediately available. In assigning this acuity, the nurse should consider that the patient may need multiple diagnostic studies or procedures and should be monitored for changes in condition while waiting.

Level 4—Semi-urgent: This category is low risk for deterioration while the patient is waiting. Symptoms are less severe and the patient can safely wait for treatment. Each facility should determine acceptable waiting times if a room is not immediately available. In assigning this acuity, the nurse should consider that the patient may need a simple diagnostic study or procedure. Patients should be reassessed while waiting, per facility protocol. To enhance customer service, the nurse should offer comfort measures.

Level 5—Nonurgent: This category is a lower risk for further deterioration while the patient is waiting. Generally, this category of patient could be seen in a lower acuity treatment area and can safely wait. Each facility should determine acceptable waiting times if a room is not immediately available. In assigning this acuity, the nurse should consider that the patient may need only a simple examination. To improve customer service, the nurse should reassess the waiting patient, per facility protocol, and offer comfort measures.

Nursing Considerations: In addition to assigning acuity based on symptoms and resources needed, the nurse is prompted when appropriate to initiate certain nursing interventions. Nurses should initiate only those nursing interventions that have been approved by their facilities.

Relevant Protocols: This section lists additional protocols to consider that may assist in determining a more appropriate patient disposition.

Appendices

This all-inclusive manual not only provides protocols to assist in daily triage activities but also includes appendices that provide essential information to help ensure that the nurses are trained in all aspects of the triage process. The appendices are as follows:

A: Triage Program Development
B: Key Questions to Ask Triage Nurses
C: Triage Pearls
D: Triage Training Outline

E: Triage Training Exercises
F: Triage Assessment Skills Checklist
G: Chart Audit Tool
H: Triage Log
I: Differential Assessment of Abdominal Pain
J: Differential Assessment of Chest Pain
K: Headache: Common Characteristics
L: MVA Triage Questions
M: Mechanisms of Injury: Adult
N: Mechanisms of Injury: School Age and Adolescent (7–17 years old)
O: Mechanisms of Injury: Toddler and Preschooler (1–6 years old)
P: Mechanisms of Injury: Infant (birth to 1 year old)
Q: Drugs of Abuse
R: Poisonings
S: Biological Agents/Chemical Agents
T: Communicable Diseases, Colds Versus Flu, and Sexually
Transmitted Diseases

Julie K. Briggs
Valerie Aarne Grossman

ACKNOWLEDGMENTS

It has been an absolute pleasure working with Valerie again on the revision of *Emergency Nursing: 5-Tier Triage Protocols*, Second Edition. I truly appreciate how hard Valerie has worked on this, her friendship, and the tenacity in moving forward with this project in spite of many conflicting priorities in our personal and professional lives. I want to express my gratitude to Elizabeth Nieginski, whose belief in us helped to pave the way for this worthwhile project. Additionally, I want to thank my husband, Worth, and my family and friends for their support and understanding of the time-consuming nature of this project.

Julie K. Briggs

I am honored to have worked on this second edition with Julie, who has been a friend and mentor for many years. I am sincerely grateful for our Springer editor Elizabeth Nieginski, who is a true supporter of nurse authors and the role we play in our profession. My deepest appreciation goes to my daughters (Sarah and Nicole), my Dad (John), and my family, friends, and colleagues who support my passion for nursing and for nurses, and I am honored each time patients allow me to help them on their journey through the healthcare system.

Valerie Aarne Grossman

Abdominal Pain, Adult

KEY QUESTIONS:

Name • Age • Onset • Allergies • Prior History • Associated Symptoms • Pain Scale • Description and Location of the Pain • Vital Signs • Medications • Exposure (Infection, Chemical, Drug) • Date of Last Menses • Gender Identification

ACUITY LEVEL/ASSESSMENT	NURSING CONSIDERATIONS
Level 1: Critical	**Resuscitation**
Pale, diaphoretic, and confused or weak Unresponsive Apnea or severe respiratory distress Pulseless	**Refer for immediate treatment** Many resources needed Staff at bedside Mobilization of resuscitation team
Level 2: High Risk	**Emergent**
Penetrating wound to abdomen New-onset, rapidly increasing pain in abdomen radiating to back or legs and age >50 years Vomiting large amount of blood Lightheadedness Sudden-onset severe pain and abnormal vital signs Signs and symptoms of dehydration Toxic substance exposure Age >50 years and systolic BP <100 mmHg Bloody stools (unrelated to hemorrhoids or rectal fissure) Vaginal bleeding saturating more than three regular-size pads per hour Abdominal pain radiates to shoulder and menses >4 weeks late History of fainting episodes Altered mental status At least two SIRS criteria: temperature >38.0°C or <36.0°C, HR >90, RR >20	**Do not delay treatment** Notify physician Nothing by mouth until examined Do not remove protruding object if present Multiple diagnostic studies or procedures Frequent consultation Constant monitoring

(continued)

Level 3: Moderate Risk	Urgent
Severe pain Heavy vaginal bleeding and possibility of pregnancy Sudden onset Constipation and fever >101°F (38.3°C) Vomiting dark, coffee-ground–like emesis Vomiting and abdominal distention Pregnancy Rapidly increasing pain Right lower quadrant pain with poor appetite, nausea or vomiting, or fever Ingestion of plant, drug, or chemical Age >65 years	**Refer for treatment as soon as possible** Nothing by mouth until examined Monitor for change in condition May need multiple diagnostic studies or procedures If vital signs abnormal, consider Level 2
Level 4: Low Risk	Semi-Urgent
Black tarry stools with foul odor History of recent abdominal surgery or chronic pain Nausea and vomiting Fever >101°F (38.3°C) Continuous pain >1 hour Painful or difficult urination Blood in urine Unexplained progressive abdominal swelling	Reassess while waiting, per facility protocol Nothing by mouth until examined Offer comfort measures May need simple diagnostic study or procedure
Level 5: Lower Risk	Nonurgent
No other symptoms, but parent/patient concerned Intermittent pain Overconsumption of foods or fluids Flatulence Sensation of bladder fullness	Reassess while waiting, per facility protocol Offer comfort measures May need examination only

RELATED PROTOCOLS:
Alcohol and Drug Use, Abuse, Overdose, and Dependence • Diarrhea, Adult • Foreign Body, Ingested • Menstrual Problems • Poisoning, Exposure or Ingestion • Pregnancy, Abdominal Pain • Urination Problems • Vaginal Bleeding, Abnormal • Vomiting

See Appendix I: Differential Assessment of Abdominal Pain

NOTES

_____

_____

_____

Abdominal Pain, Pediatric

KEY QUESTIONS:

Name • Age • Onset • Allergies • Prior History • Associated Symptoms • Pain Scale • Description and Location of the Pain • Vital Signs • Medications • Ingestion • Exposure (Infection, Chemical, Drug) • Date of Last Menses

ACUITY LEVEL/ASSESSMENT	NURSING CONSIDERATIONS
Level 1: Critical	**Resuscitation**
Pale, diaphoretic, and confused, weak, or limp Apnea or severe respiratory distress Unresponsive Pulseless	**Refer for immediate treatment** Many resources needed Staff at bedside Mobilization of resuscitation team
Level 2: High Risk	**Emergent**
Altered mental status New-onset, rapidly increasing severe pain Grasping abdomen, walking bent over, screaming, or lying with knees drawn toward chest Ingestion of unknown chemical substance, plant, medication, or object Signs and symptoms of dehydration Penetrating wound to abdomen Severe pain >1 hour	**Do not delay treatment** Notify physician Do not remove protruding object if present Multiple diagnostic studies or procedures Frequent consultation Continuous monitoring Nothing by mouth until examined
Level 3: Moderate Risk	**Urgent**
Possibility of pregnancy Sudden onset Fever >101°F (38.3°C) Age <2 years and intermittent pain Recent abdominal trauma	**Refer for treatment as soon as possible** May need multiple diagnostic studies or procedures Monitor for change in condition Nothing by mouth until examined

(continued)

Level 3: Moderate Risk (*continued*)	Urgent
Right lower quadrant pain with poor appetite, nausea, vomiting, or fever Severe nausea or vomiting Bloody or jelly-like stools Black stools History of recent abdominal surgery Unable to comfort Suspected abuse	If vital signs abnormal, consider Level 2
Level 4: Low Risk	Semi-Urgent
Mild nausea and vomiting Painful or difficult urination Blood in urine	Reassess while waiting, per facility protocol Offer comfort measures Nothing by mouth until examined May need simple diagnostic study or procedure
Level 5: Lower Risk	Nonurgent
Intermittent pain associated with eating, empty stomach, or use of pain, antibiotic, or anti-inflammatory medications Unexplained progressive abdominal swelling	Reassess while waiting, per facility protocol May need examination only Offer comfort measures

RELATED PROTOCOLS:
Alcohol and Drug Use, Abuse, Overdose, and Dependence • Diarrhea, Pediatric • Foreign Body, Ingested • Menstrual Problems • Poisoning, Exposure or Ingestion • Pregnancy, Abdominal Pain • Urination Problems • Vaginal Bleeding, Abnormal • Vomiting

See Appendices I: Differential Assessment of Abdominal Pain; N: Mechanisms of Injury: School Age and Adolescent (7–17 years old); O: Mechanisms of Injury: Toddler and Preschooler (1–6 years old); P: Mechanisms of Injury: Infant (birth to 1 year old)

NOTES

_____

_____

_____

_____

_____

Alcohol and Drug Use, Abuse, Overdose, and Dependence

KEY QUESTIONS:

Name • Age • Onset • Allergies • Prior History • Medications • Pain Scale • Vital Signs • Drug or Drinking Habits • Amount and Frequency • Hours or Days Since Last Use or Drink

ACUITY LEVEL/ASSESSMENT	NURSING CONSIDERATIONS
Level 1: Critical	**Resuscitation**
Apnea or severe difficulty breathing Pale, diaphoretic, and lightheaded or weak Unresponsive Pulseless	**Refer for immediate treatment** Many resources needed Staff at bedside Mobilization of resuscitation team
Level 2: High Risk	**Emergent**
Under the influence and rapid heart rate, chest pain, difficulty breathing, shakiness, dizziness Threat to hurt self or others Suicidal behavior Overdose Altered mental status	**Do not delay treatment** Notify physician Multiple diagnostic studies or procedures Frequent consultation Continuous monitoring Keep suicidal patient under observation
Level 3: Moderate Risk	**Urgent**
Palpitations Signs of withdrawal, rapid heartbeat, diaphoresis, fever, auditory or visual hallucinations or delusions Extremely anxious, sense of terror, agitation Severe pain New onset of hallucinations or paranoia Suicidal thoughts but no action	**Refer for treatment as soon as possible** Contact crisis worker, per facility policy Monitor for change in condition May need multiple diagnostic studies or procedures If abnormal vital signs, consider Level 2 Keep suicidal patient under observation

(continued)

Level 4: Low Risk	Semi-Urgent
Hyperventilation Profuse sweating Acute anxiety Distorted perceptions Difficulty functioning	Reassess while waiting, per facility protocol Provide bag and hyperventilation instructions as necessary Offer comfort measures May need a simple diagnostic study or procedure Maintain visual contact of patient
Level 5: Lower Risk	Nonurgent
No physical symptoms History of intermittent use and parent wants patient tested Request for help with addiction	Reassess while waiting, per facility protocol Offer comfort measures May need an examination only May need social worker consult

RELATED PROTOCOLS:
Altered Mental Status • Anxiety • Chest Pain • Diarrhea, Adult • Diarrhea, Pediatric • Vomiting
See Appendix Q: Drugs of Abuse

NOTES

_____

_____

_____

_____

_____

_____

_____

_____

_____

_____

_____

_____

_____

_____

Allergic Reaction

Name • Age • Onset • Allergies • Prior History • Severity • Pain Scale • Suspected Cause • Vital Signs • Oxygen Saturation • Medications • Recent Contrast Media

ACUITY LEVEL/ASSESSMENT	NURSING CONSIDERATIONS
Level 1: Critical	**Resuscitation**
Severe difficulty breathing Unresponsive Pale, diaphoretic, lightheaded, or weak Unable to speak Severe swelling of tongue or throat Hypotension Oxygen saturation <90% with oxygen	**Refer for immediate treatment** Staff at bedside Mobilization of resuscitation team Many resources needed
Level 2: High Risk	**Emergent**
Moderate oral swelling Audible stridor or wheezing Hoarse voice Moderate respiratory distress Speaking in short words Prior anaphylaxis requiring epinephrine Difficulty swallowing Chest pain Rapid progression of symptoms Altered mental status Urticaria and hives throughout body Oxygen saturation <94% with oxygen Oxygen saturation <90% on room air	**Do not delay treatment** Notify physician Multiple diagnostic studies or procedures Frequent consultation Continuous monitoring

(continued)

Level 3: Moderate Risk	Urgent
Symptoms persist after administration of diphenhydramine or epinephrine Minimal oral swelling Mild respiratory distress Speaking in partial sentences Persistent nausea, vomiting, or diarrhea Urticaria >50% of body Fever or severe pain	**Refer for treatment as soon as possible** Monitor for change in condition May need a breathing treatment while waiting May need multiple diagnostic studies or procedures If vital signs abnormal, consider Level 2
Level 4: Low Risk	**Semi-Urgent**
Dermal contact with allergen Speaking in full sentences Urticaria in large localized area Moderate pain	Reassess while waiting, per facility protocol Offer comfort measures May need a simple diagnostic study or procedure
Level 5: Lower Risk	**Nonurgent**
Persistent rash No respiratory problems Suspect medication reaction Urticaria in small localized area Minimal swelling in face or extremities	Reassess while waiting, per facility protocol Offer comfort measures May need an examination only

RELATED PROTOCOLS:
Asthma • Bee Sting • Breathing Problems • Hives • Rash, Adult and Pediatric

NOTES

_____

_____

_____

_____

_____

_____

_____

_____

_____

_____

Altered Mental Status

KEY QUESTIONS:
Name • Age • Onset • Allergies • Medications • Prior History • Severity • Pain Scale • Vital Signs • Oxygen Saturation • Drug Use • Chemical Exposure • Head Trauma • Signs of Stroke

ACUITY LEVEL/ASSESSMENT	NURSING CONSIDERATIONS
Level 1: Critical	**Resuscitation**
Apnea or severe respiratory distress Unresponsive Pale, diaphoretic, and lightheaded or weak Status epilepticus Pulseless Signs of stroke	**Refer for immediate treatment** Staff at bedside Mobilization of resuscitation team Many resources needed
Level 2: High Risk	**Emergent**
Altered mental status Drug or alcohol overdose Danger to self or others Severe headache Chest pain Rapid heartbeat with syncope/diaphoresis Abnormal vital signs (HR <50 or >100, RR <8) Diabetic Pregnancy and heavy vaginal bleeding or abdominal pain Severe abdominal pain Loss of movement in arms or legs, confusion, difficulty speaking, numbness or tingling, or blurred vision, and onset <2 hours ago Extreme agitation or restlessness Headache and projectile vomiting Headache, fever, and stiff or painful neck Child's body is rigid or flaccid Hallucinations, delusions, or mania	**Do not delay treatment** Notify physician Multiple diagnostic studies or procedures Frequent consultation Continuous monitoring

(continued)

Level 3: Moderate Risk	Urgent
Person is arousable, oriented, and has any of the following: headache, fever without stiff or painful neck Recent head injury or trauma (rule out head bleed) New seizure and prolonged postictal state Persistent high fever Severe abdominal pain and normal vital signs Temporary slurred speech or weakened grips Tonic or clonic seizure Recently ingested pain, cold, or sleeping medication Signs of withdrawal, rapid heartbeat, diaphoresis, fever, auditory or visual hallucinations or delusions	**Refer for treatment as soon as possible** May need multiple diagnostic studies or procedures Monitor for change in condition If vital signs abnormal, consider Level 2
Level 4: Low Risk	**Semi-Urgent**
Brief period of loss of consciousness Alcohol intoxication Recreational drug use	Reassess while waiting, per facility protocol Offer comfort measures May need simple diagnostic study or procedure
Level 5: Lower Risk	**Nonurgent**
Exhaustion Sleep deprivation	Reassess while waiting, per facility protocol Offer comfort measures May need examination only

RELATED PROTOCOLS:
Alcohol and Drug Use, Abuse, Overdose, and Dependence • Breathing Problems • Chest Pain • Fever • Headache • Head Injury •Stroke

NOTES

_____

_____

_____

_____

_____

_____

_____

Altered Mental Status

Ankle Pain and Swelling

(nontraumatic; for injury, see Extremity Injury)

KEY QUESTIONS:

Name • Age • Onset • Allergies • Prior History • Severity • Pain Scale • Vital Signs • Injury

ACUITY LEVEL/ASSESSMENT	NURSING CONSIDERATIONS
Level 1: Critical	**Resuscitation**
Ankle swelling and severe difficulty breathing	**Refer for immediate treatment** Staff at bedside Mobilization of resuscitation team Many resources needed
Level 2: High Risk	**Emergent**
Chest pain Coughing blood New onset and unable to walk No pedal pulse in affected extremity Foot pale, cold, or blue compared to other foot Severe pain Altered mental status	**Do not delay treatment** Notify physician Multiple diagnostic studies or procedures Frequent consultation Continuous monitoring
Level 3: Moderate Risk	**Urgent**
Swelling and pain in ankle, thigh, or calf Pain or swelling and fever Area over ankle, calf, or thigh hot/warm to touch or red Sudden swelling and tenderness in single leg or ankle Foot numb compared to other foot Difficulty walking Pregnancy and sudden weight gain	**Refer for treatment as soon as possible** Monitor for change in condition May need multiple diagnostic studies or procedures If vital signs abnormal, consider Level 2

(continued)

Level 4: Low Risk	Semi-Urgent
Pain in the joint or base of the big toe Red and shiny skin over the joint	Reassess while waiting, per facility protocol Offer comfort measures May need a simple diagnostic study or procedure
Level 5: Lower Risk	Nonurgent
Pregnancy and gradual weight gain	Reassess while waiting, per facility protocol Offer comfort measures May need an examination only

RELATED PROTOCOLS:
Extremity Injury

NOTES

_____

_____

_____

_____

_____

_____

_____

_____

_____

_____

_____

_____

_____

_____

_____

_____

_____

_____

_____

Anxiety

(If chest pain is present, see Chest Pain)

KEY QUESTIONS:

Name • Age • Onset • Allergies • Prior History • Medications • Severity • Pain Scale • Vital Signs • Precipitating Event

ACUITY LEVEL/ASSESSMENT	NURSING CONSIDERATIONS
Level 1: Critical	**Resuscitation**
Severe difficulty breathing Pale, diaphoretic, and lightheaded or weak	**Refer for immediate treatment** Many resources needed Staff at bedside Mobilization of resuscitation team
Level 2: High Risk	**Emergent**
New onset of hallucinations or paranoia Confusion Suicidal ideation or behavior Overdose Altered mental status	**Do not delay treatment** Notify physician Multiple diagnostic studies or procedures Frequent consultation Continuous monitoring
Level 3: Moderate Risk	**Urgent**
Palpitations Difficulty functioning Extremely anxious Severe pain	**Refer for treatment as soon as possible** Contact crisis worker, per facility policy Monitor for change in condition May need multiple diagnostic studies or procedures If abnormal vital signs, consider Level 2
Level 4: Low Risk	**Semi-Urgent**
Hyperventilation Profuse sweating Persistent upset stomach Emotional or situational stress Increased caffeine consumption	Reassess while waiting, per facility protocol Provide bag and hyperventilation instructions as necessary Offer comfort measures May need a simple diagnostic study or procedure

(continued)

Level 5: Lower Risk	Nonurgent
No physical symptoms History of anxiety episodes and now asymptomatic	Reassess while waiting, per facility protocol Offer comfort measures May need an examination only

RELATED PROTOCOLS:
Alcohol and Drug Use, Abuse, Overdose, and Dependence • Breathing Problems • Chest Pain

NOTES

_____

_____

_____

_____

_____

_____

_____

_____

_____

_____

_____

_____

_____

_____

_____

_____

_____

_____

_____

_____

_____

_____

_____

Asthma

KEY QUESTIONS:

Name • Age • Onset • Allergies • Prior Asthma History • Severity • Duration • Prior Treatment • Medications • Pain Scale • Vital Signs • Oxygen Saturation • Peak Flow Meter Measurement

ACUITY LEVEL/ASSESSMENT	NURSING CONSIDERATIONS
Level 1: Critical	**Resuscitation**
Apnea or severe respiratory distress Unable to speak Central cyanosis Unresponsive Pale, diaphoretic, lightheaded, or weak Oxygen saturation <90% with oxygen	**Refer for immediate treatment** Staff at bedside Mobilization of resuscitation team Many resources needed
Level 2: High Risk	**Emergent**
Speaking in short words Use of accessory muscles and fatigue Sudden onset of wheezing after medication, food, bee sting, or exposure to known allergen Peak flow rate <50% of baseline Altered mental status Chest pain Oxygen saturation <94% with oxygen Oxygen saturation <90% on room air Heightened anxiety, fear, or restlessness	**Do not delay treatment** Notify physician Multiple diagnostic studies or procedures Frequent consultation Continuous monitoring
Level 3: Moderate Risk	**Urgent**
Speaking in partial sentences Severe cough Prior hospitalization for same symptoms Persistent, audible wheezing 20 minutes after treatment Fever >103°F (39.4°C)	**Refer for treatment as soon as possible** Monitor for change in condition May need a breathing treatment while waiting May need multiple diagnostic studies or procedures If abnormal vital signs, consider Level 2

(continued)

Level 4: Low Risk	Semi-Urgent
Speaking in full sentences Persistent cough after use of inhaler or nebulizer Fever <103°F (39.4°C) Age >60 years and fever >101°F (38.3°C) Peak flow rate >80% of baseline	Reassess while waiting, per facility protocol Offer comfort measures May need a simple diagnostic study or procedure
Level 5: Lower Risk	Nonurgent
Fever and green or yellow nasal discharge Resolution of wheezing after use of inhaler or nebulizer Peak flow back to baseline	Reassess while waiting, per facility protocol Offer comfort measures May need an examination only

RELATED PROTOCOLS:
Allergic Reaction • Breathing Problems • Cough

NOTES

_____

_____

_____

_____

_____

_____

_____

_____

_____

_____

_____

_____

_____

_____

_____

_____

_____

_____

_____

Back Pain

KEY QUESTIONS:

Name • Age • Onset • Allergies • Prior History • Severity • Pain Scale • Vital Signs • Medications • Recent Injury or Accident

ACUITY LEVEL/ASSESSMENT	NURSING CONSIDERATIONS
Level 1: Critical	**Resuscitation**
Apnea or severe respiratory distress Unresponsive Pulseless Pale, diaphoretic, and lightheaded or weak Recent trauma and unable to move toes or severe weakness in one or both lower extremities	**Refer for immediate treatment** Staff at bedside Mobilization of resuscitation team Many resources needed
Level 2: High Risk	**Emergent**
Altered mental status New-onset, rapidly increasing pain and age >60 years New-onset loss of sensation to lower extremities Progressive weakness in legs Loss of bladder or bowel control Penetrating trauma to back or flank	**Refer for treatment within minutes** Notify physician Multiple diagnostic studies or procedures Frequent consultation Continuous monitoring Do not remove penetrating object
Level 3: Moderate Risk	**Urgent**
Severe back or abdominal pain New-onset numbness and tingling in legs Hematuria and severe abdominal or flank pain Hematuria and blunt trauma to the back or flank Pain with urination and fever >100.5°F (38.1°C) or chills New-onset, rapidly increasing pain and age <60 years	**Refer for treatment as soon as possible** Monitor for change in condition May need multiple diagnostic studies or procedures If abnormal vital signs, consider Level 2

(continued)

Level 3: Moderate Risk (*continued*)	Urgent
History of diabetes, immunosuppression, or intravenous drug abuse Unable to urinate >8 hours Male with fever and nausea or vomiting History of disc injury or back surgery	
Level 4: Low Risk	**Semi-Urgent**
Trauma within past week and worsening pain, numbness, tingling, or weakness in extremity Pain restricting ability to walk Pain increasing with activity Pain radiating to buttocks or hips	Reassess while waiting, per facility protocol Offer comfort measures May need simple diagnostic study or procedure
Level 5: Lower Risk	**Nonurgent**
Chronic low back pain Minor discomfort Rash over the painful area	Reassess while waiting, per facility protocol Offer comfort measures May need an examination only

RELATED PROTOCOLS:
Neck Pain • Traumatic Injury • Urination Problems

NOTES

_____

_____

_____

_____

_____

_____

_____

_____

_____

_____

_____

_____

Bee Sting

KEY QUESTIONS:

Name ● Age ● Onset ● Allergies ● Prior History ● Severity ● Pain Scale ● Vital Signs ● Oxygen Saturation ● Previous Bee Sting Reaction and Treatment

ACUITY LEVEL/ASSESSMENT	NURSING CONSIDERATIONS
Level 1: Critical	**Resuscitation**
Apnea or severe difficulty breathing Unresponsive Pale, diaphoretic, and lightheaded or weak Hypotension Unable to speak Severe swelling of tongue or throat Oxygen saturation <90% with oxygen	**Refer for immediate treatment** Staff at bedside Mobilization of resuscitation team Many resources needed
Level 2: High Risk	**Emergent**
Moderate oral swelling Audible stridor or wheezing Hoarse voice Moderate respiratory distress Speaking in short sentences Prior anaphylaxis requiring epinephrine Difficulty swallowing Chest pain Rapid progression of symptoms Altered mental status Urticaria and hives throughout body Bee sting in the mouth Oxygen saturation <94% with oxygen Oxygen saturation <90% on room air	**Do not delay treatment** Notify physician Multiple diagnostic studies or procedures Frequent consultation Continuous monitoring

(continued)

Level 3: Moderate Risk	Urgent
Speaking in partial sentences Nausea, vomiting, or weakness More than 10 stings Generalized hives after diphenhydramine or epinephrine Mild wheezing Minimal reaction to bee sting, and Prior anaphylaxis requiring epinephrine Bee sting in the mouth	**Refer for treatment as soon as possible** Monitor for changes in condition May need multiple diagnostic studies or procedures If abnormal vital signs, consider Level 2
Level 4: Low Risk	Semi-Urgent
Able to speak in full sentences Rash locations other than sting site Signs of infection: drainage, fever, red streaks, or pus 24-48 hours after the sting	Reassess while waiting, per facility protocol Offer comfort measures May need a simple diagnostic study or procedure
Level 5: Lower Risk	Nonurgent
Localized swelling, pain, or urticaria around sting site	Reassess while waiting, per facility protocol Offer comfort measures May need an examination only

RELATED PROTOCOLS:
Allergic Reaction • Bites, Insect and Tick • Breathing Problems • Hives

NOTES

_____

_____

_____

_____

_____

_____

_____

_____

_____

_____

Bites, Animal and Human

KEY QUESTIONS:

Name • Age • Onset • Location • Allergies • Prior History • Severity • Pain Scale • Vital Signs • Tetanus Immunization Status • Domestic Versus Wild Animal

ACUITY LEVEL/ASSESSMENT	NURSING CONSIDERATIONS
Level 1: Critical	**Resuscitation**
Apnea or severe respiratory distress Pulseless Unresponsive	**Refer for immediate treatment** Many resources needed Staff at bedside Mobilization of resuscitation team
Level 2: High Risk	**Emergent**
Altered mental status Pulsatile bleeding Multiple gaping wounds Difficulty breathing or swallowing	**Do not delay treatment** Notify physician Multiple diagnostic studies or procedures Frequent consultation Constant monitoring
Level 3: Moderate Risk	**Urgent**
Severe pain Gaping wounds	**Refer for treatment as soon as possible** May need multiple diagnostic studies or procedures Monitor for changes in condition If vital signs abnormal, consider Level 2

(continued)

Level 4: Low Risk	Semi-Urgent
Moderate pain Stable wounds Abrasive wounds Signs of infection: drainage, fever, red streaks, or pus for longer than 24 hours after the bite History of chronic illness Controlled bleeding Risk for rabies exposure	Reassess while waiting, per facility protocol Offer comfort measures May need a simple diagnostic study or procedure
Level 5: Lower Risk	**Nonurgent**
No break in skin Tetanus status unknown or booster more than 5 years ago	Reassess while waiting, per facility protocol Offer comfort measures May need examination only

RELATED PROTOCOLS:
Laceration • Puncture Wound • Wound Infection

NOTES

_____

_____

_____

_____

_____

_____

_____

_____

_____

_____

_____

_____

_____

_____

_____

_____

Bites, Insect and Tick

KEY QUESTIONS:
Name • Age • Onset • Location • Allergies • Prior History • Severity • Pain Scale • Vital Signs • Type of Insect

ACUITY LEVEL/ASSESSMENT	NURSING CONSIDERATIONS
Level 1: Critical	**Resuscitation**
Apnea or severe respiratory distress Pulseless Unresponsive Hypotension Unable to speak Severe swelling of tongue or throat Unable to swallow, drooling	**Refer for immediate treatment** Many resources needed Staff at bedside Mobilization of resuscitation team
Level 2: High Risk	**Emergent**
Altered mental status Speaking in short words Difficulty breathing or chest pain Swelling of tongue or mouth with difficulty swallowing Urticaria and hives throughout body	**Do not delay treatment** Notify physician Multiple diagnostic studies or procedures Frequent consultation Constant monitoring
Level 3: Moderate Risk	**Urgent**
Severe pain Speaking in partial sentences Prior anaphylaxis to insect bite requiring epinephrine Widespread hives Numerous bites, stings, or ticks Flu-like symptoms with a history of tick bite 2–4 weeks previously Brown recluse spider bite Black widow spider bite and no other symptoms	**Refer for treatment as soon as possible** May need multiple diagnostic studies or procedures Monitor for changes in condition If vital signs abnormal, consider Level 2

(continued)

Level 4: Low Risk	Semi-Urgent
Moderate pain Signs of infection: fever, red streaks, pus, or drainage for longer than 24 hours after bite Unable to remove tick or tick head remains under skin Peeling skin around the site	Reassess while waiting, per facility protocol Offer comfort measures May need a simple diagnostic study or procedure
Level 5: Lower Risk	Nonurgent
Sporadic hives	Reassess while waiting, per facility protocol Offer comfort measures May need examination only

RELATED PROTOCOLS:
Allergic Reaction • Laceration • Wound Infection

NOTES

_____

_____

_____

_____

_____

_____

_____

_____

_____

_____

_____

_____

_____

_____

_____

_____

_____

_____

_____

Bites, Marine Animal

KEY QUESTIONS:
Name • Age • Onset • Allergies • Prior History • Severity • Pain Scale • Vital Signs • Tetanus Immunization Status • Marine Animal Identification

ACUITY LEVEL/ASSESSMENT	NURSING CONSIDERATIONS
Level 1: Critical	**Resuscitation**
Apnea or severe difficulty breathing Unresponsive Pale, diaphoretic, and lightheaded or weak Hypotension Unable to speak	**Refer for immediate treatment** Staff at bedside Mobilization of resuscitation team Many resources needed
Level 2: High Risk	**Emergent**
Altered mental status Pulsatile bleeding Limb amputation Chest pain or difficulty breathing Swelling of throat, tongue, lips Loss of pulses distal to injury	**Do not delay treatment** Notify physician Multiple diagnostic studies or procedures Frequent consultation Continuous monitoring
Level 3: Moderate Risk	**Urgent**
Severe pain Diaphoretic Pallor Hives Extremity swelling Vision changes Prior anaphylaxis requiring epinephrine	**Refer for treatment as soon as possible** Monitor for changes in condition May need multiple diagnostic studies or procedures If abnormal vital signs, consider Level 2

(continued)

Level 4: Low Risk	Semi-Urgent
Moderate pain Stung by Portuguese man-of-war jellyfish Decreased range of motion Stinger present	Reassess while waiting, per facility protocol Offer comfort measures For catfish, lionfish, scorpionfish, sea urchin, stingrays, starfish, stonefish, and surgeon-fish spine punctures, consider soaking injured part in hot saltwater for 30–90 minutes for pain relief while waiting May need a simple diagnostic study or procedure
Level 5: Lower Risk	Nonurgent
History of nonpoisonous bite with no signs or symptoms Tetanus status unknown or booster older than 5 years	Reassess while waiting, per facility protocol Offer comfort measures May need an examination only

RELATED PROTOCOLS:
Allergic Reaction • Laceration • Puncture Wound • Wound Infection

NOTES

_____

_____

_____

_____

_____

_____

_____

_____

_____

_____

_____

_____

_____

_____

Bites, Snake

Name • Age • Onset • Location • Allergies • Prior History • Severity • Pain Scale • Vital Signs • Oxygen Saturation • Tetanus Immunization Status • Type of Snake

ACUITY LEVEL/ASSESSMENT	NURSING CONSIDERATIONS
Level 1: Critical	**Resuscitation**
Apnea or severe difficulty breathing Unresponsive Pale, diaphoretic, and lightheaded or weak Hypotension Unable to speak Severe swelling of tongue or throat Oxygen saturation <90% with oxygen	**Refer for immediate treatment** Many resources needed Staff at bedside Mobilization of resuscitation team
Level 2: High Risk	**Emergent**
Altered mental status Bite from a poisonous snake, such as rattlesnake, copperhead, water moccasin, or coral snake Chest pain Difficulty swallowing or breathing	**Do not delay treatment** Notify physician Multiple diagnostic studies or procedures Frequent consultation Constant monitoring
Level 3: Moderate Risk	**Urgent**
Severe pain Puncture wound(s) from unidentified snake Purple rash, fever, pallor, or facial numbness or tingling Prior anaphylaxis to snake bite requiring epinephrine	**Refer for treatment as soon as possible** May need multiple diagnostic studies or procedures Monitor for change in condition If vital signs abnormal, consider Level 2

(continued)

Level 4: Low Risk	Semi-Urgent
Moderate pain Multiple bites from nonpoisonous snake Signs of local infection: drainage, fever, red streaks, or pus for longer than 24 hours after bite Swelling around the wound	Reassess while waiting, per facility protocol Offer comfort measures May need a simple diagnostic study or procedure
Level 5: Lower Risk	**Nonurgent**
Need for updated tetanus immunization	Reassess while waiting, per facility protocol Offer comfort measures May need examination only

RELATED PROTOCOLS:
Allergic Reaction • Laceration • Wound Infection

NOTES

_____

_____

_____

_____

_____

_____

_____

_____

_____

_____

_____

_____

_____

_____

_____

_____

_____

Body Art Complications

KEY QUESTIONS:

Name • Age • Onset • Allergies • Prior History (Including Infectious Diseases) • Severity • Pain Scale • Vital Signs • Oximetry • Location of Body Art • Performed by Whom (Professional vs. Amateur) • When Performed • Immunizations (Diphtheria and Tetanus [dT], Hepatitis B)

ACUITY LEVEL/ASSESSMENT	NURSING CONSIDERATIONS
Level 1: Critical	**Resuscitation**
Apnea or severe respiratory distress Pulseless Unresponsive Pale, diaphoretic, and lightheaded or weak	**Refer for immediate treatment** Staff at bedside Mobilization of resuscitation team Many resources needed Remove piercings that interfere with C-spine stabilization, intubation, Sager splint, Foley catheter, defibrillator, or imaging Avoid using wire cutters to remove piercings
Level 2: High Risk	**Emergent**
Altered mental status Fever, hypotension, tachycardia, weakness Chest pain Piercing torn from site and unable to stop bleeding with pressure	**Do not delay treatment** Notify physician Multiple diagnostic studies or procedures Frequent consultation Continuous monitoring Remove piercings that interfere with C-spine stabilization, intubation, Sager splint, Foley catheter, or defibrillation Avoid using wire cutters to remove piercings
Level 3: Moderate Risk	**Urgent**
Severe pain Skin reddened, peeling off in sheets Skin red and warm to touch and fever Fever, chills, general malaise, or headache	**Refer for treatment as soon as possible** May need multiple diagnostic studies or procedures Monitor for change in condition Leave piercing in place if possible If vital signs abnormal, consider Level 2

(continued)

Level 3: Moderate Risk (*continued*)	Urgent
Vomiting, abdominal pain, jaundice Piercing torn from site, bleeding controlled Swallowed oral jewelry Swollen lymph nodes and fever At least two SIRS criteria: temperature >38.0°C or <36.0°C; HR >90; RR >20	

Level 4: Low Risk	Semi-Urgent
Moderate pain Skin red and warm to touch, swelling, or red streaks (no fever) Jewelry slipped inside piercing site, no visible jewelry Swollen lymph node Darkened, hard, and painful area around the piercing or tattoo	Reassess while waiting, per facility protocol Offer comfort measures May need simple diagnostic study or procedure Leave piercing in place if possible

Level 5: Lower Risk	Nonurgent
Body art remorse (patient or parent requests reversal of procedure) No other symptoms, new piercing or tattoo, and patient or parent concerned	Reassess while waiting, per facility protocol Offer comfort measures May need examination only

COMMON COMPLICATIONS: BODY PIERCING

Location	Jewelry Used	Healing Time	Common Complications
Ampallang	Barbell stud	6–12 months	• Keloid formation • May interrupt the flow of urine (may need to sit to void) • Formation of abscesses, cysts, or boils • Ripping and tearing of skin if jewelry gets caught on clothing

(continued)

Location	Jewelry Used	Healing Time	Common Complications
Cheek	Labret stud	6–8 weeks	• Swelling, infection, gum injury, increased salivation • Chipped or broken teeth • Speech impairment • Aspiration or ingestion of loosened jewelry • Difficulty chewing and swallowing • Massive systemic infection, septic shock • Formation of abscesses, cysts, or boils
Clitoris	Captive bead ring, barbell stud	4–10 weeks	• Keloid formation • Formation of abscesses, cysts, or boils • Ripping and tearing of skin if jewelry gets caught on clothing
Clitoris hood	Captive bead ring, captive stone ring, circular barbell	4–10 weeks	• Keloid formation • Formation of abscesses, cysts, or boils • Ripping and tearing of skin if jewelry gets caught on clothing
Ear cartilage	Same pieces as an earlobe; larger gauge is used	4–12 months	• Keloid formation • Formation of abscesses, cysts, or boils • Prone to *Pseudomonas* infections • Ripping and tearing of skin if jewelry gets caught on clothing
Ear plug	Increasing sizes of an object	Gradual enlargement of lobe	• Keloid formation • Overstretching of skin
Earlobe	Captive bead ring, circular barbell, captive stone ring	4–6 weeks	• Keloid formation • Formation of abscesses, cysts, or boils • Ripping and tearing of skin if jewelry gets caught on clothing

(continued)

Body Art Complications

Location	Jewelry Used	Healing Time	Common Complications
Eyebrow	Captive bead ring, captive stone ring, barbell studs	6–8 weeks	• Keloid formation • Ripping and tearing of skin if jewelry gets caught on clothing • Formation of abscesses, cysts, or boils • Excess hair growth over piercing area • Development of cysts • Periorbital cellulitis
Foreskin	Captive bead ring, captive stone ring, circular barbell	6–8 weeks	• Formation of abscesses, cysts, or boils • Ripping and tearing of skin if jewelry gets caught on clothing
Frenum	Barbell stud	6–8 weeks	• Keloid formation • Formation of abscesses, cysts, or boils • Ripping and tearing of skin if jewelry gets caught on clothing
Hand web	Captive bead ring, captive stone ring, barbell studs	6–12 months	• Difficult healing, due to high rate of infection • Formation of abscesses, cysts, or boils • Ripping and tearing of skin if jewelry gets caught on clothing
Implants	Captive bead ring, captive stone ring, barbell studs, circular barbell, other assorted items (beads, spikes, coral, etc.)	2–4 months	• Pressure on nerves, blood vessels, and muscles • Radiating pain that continues after complete healing • Shifting (when the object moves from its intended place) • Rejection by the body's immune system • Excess hair growth over implantation area • Formation of abscesses, cysts, or boils

(continued)

Location	Jewelry Used	Healing Time	Common Complications
Labia majora	Captive bead ring, captive stone ring, circular barbell	6–10 weeks	• Keloid formation • Formation of abscesses, cysts, or boils • Ripping and tearing of skin if jewelry gets caught on clothing
Labia minora	Captive bead ring, captive stone ring, circular barbell	6–10 weeks	• Keloid formation • Formation of abscesses, cysts, or boils • Ripping and tearing of skin if jewelry gets caught on clothing
Lip	Captive bead ring, captive stone ring, barbell studs	2–3 months	• Swelling, infection, gingival injury, increased salivation • Keloid formation • Excess hair growth over pierced area • Chipped or broken teeth • Speech impairment • Aspiration or ingestion of loosened jewelry • Massive systemic infection, septic shock • Formation of abscesses, cysts, or boils • Ripping and tearing of skin if jewelry gets caught on clothing
Nasal septum	Captive bead ring, circular barbell, septum retainer	2–8 months	• Formation of abscesses, cysts, or boils • Ripping and tearing of skin if jewelry gets caught on clothing
Navel	Captive bead ring, captive stone ring, circular barbell	4–12 months	• Very slow to heal: redness of area can last for months • Keloid formation

(continued)

Location	Jewelry Used	Healing Time	Common Complications
Navel (*continued*)			• Excess hair growth over pierced area • Very high rate of infection (compared to other piercings) because of constant friction, rubbing, and movement • Bacteria-friendly environment (warm, dark, and moist) • Formation of abscesses, cysts, or boils • Ripping and tearing of skin if jewelry gets caught on clothing
Nipples (female)	Captive bead ring, captive stone ring, circular barbell	3–6 months	• May damage some of the milk-producing ducts, causing mastitis or problems with future breastfeeding • Formation of abscesses, cysts, or boils • Ripping and tearing of skin if jewelry gets caught on clothing
Nipples (male)	Captive bead ring, captive stone ring, circular barbell	3–6 months	• Formation of abscesses, cysts, or boils • Ripping and tearing of skin if jewelry gets caught on clothing
Nostril	Captive bead ring, captive stone ring	2–4 months	• Keloid formation • Formation of abscesses, cysts, or boils • Ripping and tearing of skin if jewelry gets caught on clothing
Scrotum	Captive bead ring, captive stone ring, circular barbell	6–8 weeks	• Ripping and tearing of skin if jewelry gets caught on clothing

(*continued*)

Location	Jewelry Used	Healing Time	Common Complications
Tongue	Barbell stud	4-6 weeks	• Swelling, infection, gingival injury, increased salivation • Keloid formation • Chipped or broken teeth • Speech impairment • Aspiration or ingestion of loosened jewelry • Difficulty breathing, chewing, and swallowing • Prolonged bleeding • Massive systemic infection, septic shock • Damage to veins and nerves, including neuroma development
Tragus	Captive bead ring, circular barbell, captive stone ring	6-12 months	• Formation of abscesses, cysts, or boils
Uvula	Captive bead ring, circular barbell, barbell stud	6-8 weeks	• Swelling, infection, injury, increased salivation • Speech impairment • Aspiration or ingestion of loosened jewelry • Difficulty breathing and swallowing • Formation of abscesses, cysts, or boils

RELATED PROTOCOLS:
Laceration • Wound Infection

NOTES

_____

_____

_____

_____

_____

Breast Problems

KEY QUESTIONS:
Name • Age • Onset • Allergies • Prior History • Severity • Pain Scale • Vital Signs • Gender Identification

ACUITY LEVEL/ASSESSMENT	NURSING CONSIDERATIONS
Level 1: Critical	**Resuscitation**
Apnea or severe respiratory distress Unresponsive Pale, diaphoretic, and lightheaded or weak Hypotension	**Refer for immediate treatment** Many resources needed Staff at bedside Mobilization of resuscitation team
Level 2: High Risk	**Emergent**
Altered mental status Difficulty breathing or chest pain	**Do not delay treatment** Notify physician Multiple diagnostic studies or procedures Frequent consultation Constant monitoring
Level 3: Moderate Risk	**Urgent**
Severe pain Gaping lacerations	**Refer for treatment as soon as possible** May need multiple diagnostic studies or procedures Monitor for changes in condition If vital signs abnormal, consider Level 2

(continued)

Level 4: Low Risk	Semi-Urgent
Moderate pain Skin ulceration Bloody discharge Foul-smelling discharge from nipples Red, swollen, hot breasts Trauma to breast Signs of infection: drainage, fever, red streaks, or pus	Reassess while waiting, per facility protocol Offer comfort measures May need a simple diagnostic study or procedure
Level 5: Lower Risk	Nonurgent
Nipple discharge in nonpregnant woman Lump in breast unrelated to menstrual cycle Dimpling of breast tissue Lump in a male breast Unable to remove piercing	Reassess while waiting, per facility protocol Offer comfort measures May need examination only

RELATED PROTOCOLS:
Body Art Complications • Lacerations • Wound Infection

NOTES

_____

_____

_____

_____

_____

_____

_____

_____

_____

_____

_____

_____

_____

_____

_____

_____

Breathing Problems

KEY QUESTIONS:

Name • Age • Weight • Onset • Allergies • Prior History • Severity • Vital Signs • Oxygen Saturation • Medications • Pain Scale

ACUITY LEVEL/ASSESSMENT	NURSING CONSIDERATIONS
Level 1: Critical	**Resuscitation**
Apnea or severe respiratory distress Unresponsive Pulseless Unable to speak Central cyanosis Oxygen saturation <90% with oxygen Severe retractions or acute cyanosis (pediatric)	**Refer for immediate treatment** Staff at bedside Mobilization of resuscitation team Many resources needed
Level 2: High Risk	**Emergent**
Altered mental status Feeling of suffocation History of pulmonary embolus, blood clots, or lung collapse Chest pain Speaking in short words Pale skin or cyanotic fingernails Obstructed airway Foreign body aspiration Moderate retractions (pediatric) Drooling Oxygen saturation <94% with oxygen Oxygen saturation <90% on room air Audible wheezes or severe stridor	**Do not delay treatment** Notify physician Multiple diagnostic studies or procedures Frequent consultation Continuous monitoring Accurate oxygen saturation dependent upon good circulation and warm extremities Carbon monoxide poisoning will show adequate oxygen saturation in spite of poor oxygenation

(continued)

Level 2: High Risk (*continued*)	Emergent
Diaphoresis Moderate use of accessory muscles Difficulty breathing and exposure to allergen that caused a significant reaction in the past Trauma and chest deformity At least two SIRS criteria: temperature >38.0°C or <36.0°C, HR >90, RR >20	
Level 3: Moderate Risk	**Urgent**
Pain increasing with movement or breathing Speaking in partial sentences Mild, audible wheezes at rest Tight cough Frothy pink or copious white sputum History of asthma not relieved with inhaler Sudden or progressive shortness of breath and wheezing within past 2 hours; Recent trauma, surgery, or childbirth Inhalation of a foreign body Pallor High anxiety	**Refer for treatment as soon as possible** Monitor for changes in condition May need a breathing treatment while waiting May need multiple diagnostic studies or procedures If abnormal vital signs, consider Level 2
Level 4: Low Risk	**Semi-Urgent**
Speaking in full sentences Fever >103°F (39.4°C) Productive cough with gray, green, or yellow sputum Age >60 years and fever >101°F (38.3°C)	Reassess while waiting, per facility protocol Offer comfort measures May need a simple diagnostic study or procedure
Level 5: Lower Risk	**Nonurgent**
Oxygen saturation >95% on room air Occasional nonproductive cough Hyperventilation and numbness or tingling in fingers or face New stressful event or situation Exposure to environment irritant Recent cold or flu symptoms	Reassess while waiting, per facility protocol Offer comfort measures May need an examination only

NOTES

_____

_____

_____

_____

_____

_____

_____

_____

_____

_____

_____

_____

_____

_____

_____

Burns

KEY QUESTIONS:

Name • Age • Onset • Allergies • Medications • Prior History • Mechanism of Injury • Severity • Pain Scale • Vital Signs • Last Tetanus Immunization • Size and Location of Burn

ACUITY LEVEL/ASSESSMENT	NURSING CONSIDERATIONS
Level 1: Critical	**Resuscitation**
Apnea or severe respiratory distress Pulseless Unresponsive Pale, diaphoretic, and lightheaded or weak	**Refer for immediate treatment** Staff at bedside Mobilization of resuscitation team Many resources needed
Level 2: High Risk	**Emergent**
Altered mental status Extensive white and painless burn Extensive red and blistered burn and severe pain Difficulty breathing Chest pain or rapid irregular heartbeat Electrical, chemical, thermal, or radiation burn Smoke inhalation with singed facial hair Burn circles neck or extremity (and weak/ absent distal pulse)	**Do not delay treatment** Notify physician Multiple diagnostic studies or procedures Frequent consultation Continuous monitoring
Level 3: Moderate Risk	**Urgent**
Severe pain Burned area charred (small area) Blistered or white painless burn larger than the size of a hand Burn over a joint Blisters on face or neck Burn >1 inch and on face, eyes, ears, neck, hands, feet, or genital area	**Refer for treatment as soon as possible** Reassess, per facility protocol May need multiple diagnostic studies or procedures Monitor for changes in condition If vital signs abnormal, consider Level 2

(continued)

Level 4: Low Risk	Semi-Urgent
History of chronic illness Moderate pain Signs of infection Tetanus immunization older than 5 years or immunization status unknown	Reassess while waiting, per facility protocol Offer comfort measures May need simple diagnostic study or procedure
Level 5: Lower Risk	Nonurgent
Minimal pain Multiple open blisters	Reassess while waiting, per facility protocol Offer comfort measures May need examination only

RELATED PROTOCOLS:
Breathing Problems • Laceration • Poisoning, Exposure or Ingestion • Wound Infection

NOTES

Chest Pain

KEY QUESTIONS:

Name • Age • Onset • Allergies • Prior History • Medications • Severity • Pain Scale • Associated Symptoms • Vital Signs • Oxygen Saturation • History of Pacemaker, Automatic Implantable Cardioverter-Defibrillator [AICD], Left Ventricular Assist Device [LVAD], Heart Transplant, etc.

ACUITY LEVEL/ASSESSMENT	NURSING CONSIDERATIONS
Level 1: Critical	**Resuscitation**
Apnea or severe respiratory distress Unresponsive Pulseless Central cyanosis Hypotension LVAD failure	**Refer for immediate treatment** Staff at bedside Mobilization of resuscitation team Many resources needed
Level 2: High Risk	**Emergent**
Altered mental status Lightheadedness or weakness Cool, moist skin Nausea or vomiting Pain radiates to neck, shoulders, jaw, back, or arms Age >35 years and heart palpitations Difficulty breathing Skin pale Bilateral rales or rhonchi Persistent pain after three doses of nitroglycerin 5 minutes apart Known cardiac disease Severe chest pain at rest or awakens person Coughing up blood History of recent trauma, childbirth, or surgery Overdose or drug use within past 24 hours History of heart disease, diabetes, congestive heart failure, or blood clotting problems Severe pain	**Refer for treatment within minutes** Notify physician Administer oxygen per facility protocol Obtain 12-lead EKG per facility protocol Establish IV line per facility protocol Administer aspirin per facility protocol Administer nitroglycerin per facility protocol Many diagnostic studies or procedures Frequent consultation Continuous monitoring If chest pain severe and worsens with breathing, movement, palpitation, or coughing, consider Level 1

(continued)

Level 3: Moderate Risk	Urgent
Moderate pain Stable vital signs and rhythm Age <35 years and heart palpitations No difficulty breathing Heavy smoker Pain, swelling, warmth, or redness of leg Pain with exertion Strong family history of heart disease, heart attack, stroke, or diabetes	**Refer for treatment as soon as possible** Monitor for changes in condition May need multiple diagnostic studies or procedures If abnormal vital signs, consider Level 2
Level 4: Low Risk	Semi-Urgent
Recent injury and pain increases with movement and inspiration Fever, cough, congestion	Reassess while waiting, per facility protocol Offer comfort measures May need simple diagnostic study or procedure
Level 5: Lower Risk	Nonurgent
Pain worsens when pressure applied to the area Intermittent pain increases with deep breathing and coughing Chronic pain	Reassess while waiting, per facility protocol Offer comfort measures May need examination only

RELATED PROTOCOLS:
Breathing Problems • Cold Symptoms
See Appendix J: Differential Assessment of Chest Pain

NOTES

_____

_____

_____

_____

_____

_____

_____

_____

Cold Exposure, Hypothermia/ Frostbite

KEY QUESTIONS:

Name • Age • Onset • Length and Time of Exposure • Body Temperature • Vital Signs • Pain Scale • Medications • Tetanus Status

ACUITY LEVEL/ASSESSMENT	NURSING CONSIDERATIONS
Level 1: Critical	**Resuscitation**
Apnea or severe respiratory distress Pulseless Unresponsive	**Refer for immediate treatment** Staff at bedside Mobilization of resuscitation team Many resources needed
Level 2: High Risk	**Emergent**
Altered mental status lethargy Depressed level of consciousness Muscle rigidity Skin hard, cold, white, blue, yellow, or waxy (third-degree frostbite) Purple fingers, toes, or nail beds Unable to raise body temperature Poor coordination or lightheadedness Infant, elderly, disabled, or immunosuppressed	**Do not delay treatment** Notify physician Multiple diagnostic studies or procedures Frequent consultation Continuous monitoring Rewarm as soon as possible (If exposure <24 hours, rewarm using warm IV fluids, warm wet packs, or warm water: avoid heat lamps and dry heating pads; stop rewarming when part is warm, red, and moves easily)
Level 3: Moderate Risk	**Urgent**
Severe pain Blistering or peeling skin (second-degree frostbite) Persistent shivering after warming	**Refer for treatment as soon as possible** Monitor for changes in condition May need multiple diagnostic studies or procedures If abnormal vital signs, consider Level 2

(continued)

Level 4: Low Risk	Semi-Urgent
Signs of infection (redness, swelling, pain, red streaks, warmth) Cold, mild shivering Redness followed by blister formation in 24–36 hours and skin is soft	Reassess while waiting, per facility protocol Offer comfort measures May need a simple diagnostic study or procedure
Level 5: Lower Risk	Nonurgent
Cold but no skin blistering Able to talk and drink warm fluids Asymptomatic	Reassess while waiting, per facility protocol Offer comfort measures May need an examination only

RELATED PROTOCOLS:
Confusion • Lightheadedness/Fainting

NOTES
_____
_____
_____
_____
_____
_____
_____
_____
_____
_____
_____
_____
_____
_____
_____
_____
_____
_____

Cold Symptoms

KEY QUESTIONS:

Name • Age • Onset • Allergies • Prior History • Associated Symptoms • Pain Scale • Vital Signs • Oxygen Saturation • Medications

ACUITY LEVEL/ASSESSMENT	NURSING CONSIDERATIONS
Level 1: Critical	**Resuscitation**
Apnea or severe respiratory distress Pale, diaphoretic, and lightheaded or weak Oxygen saturation <90% with oxygen	**Refer for immediate treatment** Many resources needed Staff at bedside Mobilization of resuscitation team
Level 2: High Risk	**Emergent**

Altered mental status
Difficulty breathing (unrelated to nasal congestion)
Chest pain (unrelated to chest wall movement)
Petechiae, fever, headache, pain with neck flexion
Oxygen saturation <94% with oxygen
Oxygen saturation <90% on room air
Infant <12 weeks old with a temperature
   >100.4°F (38.0°C)
	Do not delay treatment
	Notify physician
	Multiple diagnostic studies or
	   procedures
	Frequent consultation
	Constant monitoring

Level 3: Moderate Risk	**Urgent**

Severe pain
Fever >103°F (39.4°C)
Child >12 weeks of age and fever >105°F (40.5°C)
Signs of dehydration
Neck pain or rigidity
History of immunosuppression, age >60 years,
   diabetes, and fever >100.5°F (38.1°C)
Chest pain with deep inspiration or coughing
At least two SIRS criteria: temperature >38.0°C or
   <36.0°C, HR >90, RR >20
	**Refer for treatment as soon as
	possible**
	May need multiple diagnostic studies or
	   procedures
	Monitor for changes in condition
	If vital signs abnormal, consider Level 2

(continued)

Level 4: Low Risk	Semi-Urgent
Moderate pain Intermittent wheezing unrelated to diagnosed asthma History of chronic illness Sinus pain, sore throat, or fever persists >3 days Green or brown sputum >72 hours	Reassess while waiting, per facility protocol Offer comfort measures May need a simple diagnostic study or procedure
Level 5: Lower Risk	Nonurgent
Earache Sore throat Runny nose Intermittent cough	Reassess while waiting, per facility protocol Offer comfort measures May need examination only

RELATED PROTOCOLS:
Breathing Problems • Fever • Sore Throat

NOTES

_____

_____

_____

_____

_____

_____

_____

_____

_____

_____

_____

_____

_____

_____

Confusion

KEY QUESTIONS:

Name • Age • Onset • Allergies • Prior History • Severity • Pain Scale • Vital Signs

ACUITY LEVEL/ASSESSMENT	NURSING CONSIDERATIONS
Level 1: Critical	**Resuscitation**
Apnea or severe difficulty breathing Pale, diaphoretic, lightheaded, or weak Status epilepticus Hypotension Unresponsive Stroke signs and symptoms	**Refer for immediate treatment** Staff at bedside Mobilization of resuscitation team Many resources needed
Level 2: High Risk	**Emergent**
Recent head injury or trauma with loss of consciousness Drug or alcohol overdose Exposure to chemicals Ingestion of drug(s) Disoriented to name, date, or place Temperature >102°F (38.9°C) Headache, fever, and stiff or painful neck Sudden weakness on one side of the body Difficulty speaking	**Do not delay treatment** Notify physician Multiple diagnostic studies or procedures Frequent consultation Continuous monitoring
Level 3: Moderate Risk	**Urgent**
History of psychosis History of diabetes, stroke, high blood pressure, or cardiac disease Fever >101°F (38.3°C) in the elderly or immunosuppressed History of drug or alcohol abuse	**Refer for treatment as soon as possible** Monitor for changes in condition May need multiple diagnostic studies or procedures If abnormal vital signs, consider Level 2

(continued)

Level 3: Moderate Risk (*continued*)	Urgent
Signs of withdrawal: rapid heartbeat, diaphoresis, fever, auditory or visual hallucinations or delusions At least two SIRS criteria: temperature >38.0°C or <36.0°C, HR >90, RR >20	

Level 4: Low Risk	Semi-Urgent
Taking medications known to cause confusion Recently taking a new medication History of seizure disorder Persistent confusion after fever clears History of dementia or chronic brain syndrome and change in status Low-grade fever	Reassess while waiting, per facility protocol Offer comfort measures May need a simple diagnostic study or procedure

Level 5: Lower Risk	Nonurgent
History of dementia or chronic brain syndrome and no change in status Afebrile	Reassess while waiting, per facility protocol Offer comfort measures May need an examination only

RELATED PROTOCOLS:
Alcohol and Drug Use, Abuse, Overdose, and Dependence • Altered Mental Status • Fever

NOTES

_____

_____

_____

_____

_____

_____

_____

_____

_____

_____

Contusion

KEY QUESTIONS:

Name • Age • Onset • Allergies • Prior History • Severity • Pain Scale • Vital Signs • Oxygen Saturation • Specifics of Injury • Medications (Blood Thinners, Aspirin [ASA], Herbal Supplements)

ACUITY LEVEL/ASSESSMENT	NURSING CONSIDERATIONS
Level 1: Critical	**Resuscitation**
Apnea or severe respiratory distress Pulseless Unresponsive Pale, diaphoretic, and lightheaded or weak	**Refer for immediate treatment** Staff at bedside Mobilization of resuscitation team Many resources needed
Level 2: High Risk	**Emergent**
Altered mental status Chest pain Blunt trauma to chest or abdomen Chest, flank, or abdominal wall bruising Possibility of deep trauma (solid organ laceration, hollow organ rupture) Risk of domestic violence or human trafficking (separate patient from visitor for safety) History inconsistent with injuries Battle sign or raccoon eyes Circumferential ecchymoses of neck Fever, weakness, tachycardia, hypotension	**Do not delay treatment** Notify physician Multiple diagnostic studies or procedures Frequent consultation Continuous monitoring Refer to Bruise Assessment chart at end of protocol to determine age of contusion
Level 3: Moderate Risk	**Urgent**
Severe pain Trauma and possibility of a fracture or muscle hematoma Bite marks Bruising over multiple areas Difficulty walking	**Refer for treatment as soon as possible** May need multiple diagnostic studies or procedures Monitor for changes in condition Monitor circulation, movement, and sensation of affected extremity

(continued)

Level 3: Moderate Risk (*continued*)	Urgent
History of bleeding problems or use of blood thinners Increased pain, swelling, redness, fever, or red streaks	Refer to Bruise Assessment chart at end of protocol to determine age of contusion If vital signs abnormal, consider Level 2
Level 4: Low Risk	**Semi-Urgent**
Moderate pain Small bruises on extremities	Reassess while waiting, per facility protocol Offer comfort measures May need simple diagnostic study or procedure Refer to Bruise Assessment chart at end of protocol to determine age of contusion
Level 5: Lower Risk	**Nonurgent**
Contusion healing but patient or parent concerned No other symptoms	Reassess while waiting, per facility protocol Offer comfort measures May need examination only Refer to Bruise Assessment chart below to determine age of contusion

BRUISE ASSESSMENT

Color of Bruise	Age of Bruise
Red, reddish blue	<24 hours since time of injury
Dark blue, dark purple	1–4 days
Green, yellow–green	5–7 days
Yellow, brown	7–10 days
Normal tint, disappearance of bruise	1–3 weeks

RELATED PROTOCOLS:
Extremity Injury • Traumatic Injury

Cough

KEY QUESTIONS:

Name • Age • Onset • Allergies • Prior History • Severity • Pain Scale • Vital Signs • Oxygen Saturation • Medications • Associated Symptoms • Recent Travel • Exposure to Tuberculosis, Pertussis, or Other Ill People

ACUITY LEVEL/ASSESSMENT	NURSING CONSIDERATIONS
Level 1: Critical	**Resuscitation**
Apnea or severe respiratory distress Unresponsive Unable to speak Oxygen saturation <90% with oxygen Central cyanosis	**Refer for immediate treatment** Staff at bedside Mobilization of resuscitation team Many resources needed
Level 2: High Risk	**Emergent**
Altered mental status Drooling Severe difficulty breathing Intercostal and substernal retractions Severe stridor Speaking in short sentences International travel Blue lips or tongue Feeling of suffocation Frothy pink sputum Child <12 months old with rapid breathing and persistent cough At least two SIRS criteria: temperature >38.0°C or <36.0°C, HR >90, RR >20	**Do not delay treatment** Notify physician Multiple diagnostic studies or procedures Frequent consultation Continuous monitoring

(continued)

Level 3: Moderate Risk	Urgent
Severe pain Speaking in partial sentences Mild stridor Wheezing heard across the room History of asthma and nonresponsive to home care Fever >103°F (39.4°C) Fever >100.5°F (38.1°C) and age >60 years or immunosuppressed Coughing up blood Cough unrelated to cold symptoms and history of recent trauma, surgery, childbirth, heart attacks, blood clots, or long sedentary period	**Refer for treatment as soon as possible** Monitor for changes in condition May need multiple diagnostic studies or procedures If abnormal vital signs, consider Level 2
Level 4: Low Risk	Semi-Urgent
Moderate pain Speaking in full sentences No stridor Wheezing, rales, or rhonchi with auscultation History of asthma and has not taken medication or a breathing treatment Persistent fever longer than 72 hours and no response to fever-reducing measures Coughing interferes with sleep Intermittent barking cough unrelieved by exposure to cool air, humidifier, or steam Green or brown sputum for longer than 72 hours	Reassess while waiting, per facility protocol Offer comfort measures May need a simple diagnostic study or procedure
Level 5: Lower Risk	Nonurgent
History of croup Cough caused by exercise Intermittent chest discomfort with deep, productive cough No other signs or symptoms but parent or patient concerned Cough and weight loss Earache Sore throat	Reassess while waiting, per facility protocol Offer comfort measures May need an examination only

RELATED PROTOCOLS:
Asthma • Breathing Problems • Cold Symptoms

Crying Baby

KEY QUESTIONS:

Name • Age • Onset • Allergies • Prior History (Including Birth History) • Severity • Pain Scale • Vital Signs • Oxygen Saturation

ACUITY LEVEL/ASSESSMENT	NURSING CONSIDERATIONS
Level 1: Critical	**Resuscitation**
Apnea or severe respiratory distress Central cyanosis	**Refer for immediate treatment** Staff at bedside Mobilization of resuscitation team Many resources needed
Level 2: High Risk	**Emergent**
Altered mental status Temperature >100.4°F (38°C) in infants <12 weeks of age Blue lips or tongue Petechiae Extreme lethargy Bulging fontanel	**Do not delay treatment** Notify physician Multiple diagnostic studies or procedures Frequent consultation Continuous monitoring
Level 3: Moderate Risk	**Urgent**
Inability to console infant Recent trauma Risk of abuse Unexplained bruising Intermittent lethargy or irritability Persistent crying longer than 2 hours Projectile vomiting Signs of dehydration Finger or toe swollen or discolored	**Refer for treatment as soon as possible** Monitor for change in condition May need multiple diagnostic studies or procedures If abnormal vital signs, consider Level 2 If suspected abuse, keep infant under observation

(continued)

Level 4: Low Risk	Semi-Urgent
Recent use of "cold" medication Fever, vomiting, cold symptoms Raised, red, or itchy rash Fever, vomiting, or pulling ears	Reassess while waiting, per facility protocol Offer comfort measures May need a simple diagnostic study or procedure
Level 5: Lower Risk	Nonurgent
More than 2 hours since last feeding More than 3 hours since last nap Recent immunizations and fever	Reassess while waiting, per facility protocol Offer comfort measures May need an examination only

RELATED PROTOCOLS:
Sore Throat
See Appendix P: Mechanisms of Injury: Infant (birth to 1 year old)

NOTES

_____

_____

_____

_____

_____

_____

_____

_____

_____

_____

_____

_____

_____

_____

_____

_____

_____

_____

_____

Depression

KEY QUESTIONS:
Name • Age • Onset • Allergies • Prior History • Severity • Pain Scale • Vital Signs •
Medications • Recent Traumatic Event

ACUITY LEVEL/ASSESSMENT	NURSING CONSIDERATIONS
Level 1: Critical	**Resuscitation**
Severe respiratory distress Hypotension Pale, diaphoretic, and lightheaded or weak	**Refer for immediate treatment** Staff at bedside Mobilization of resuscitation team Many resources needed
Level 2: High Risk	**Emergent**
Altered mental status Suicidal or homicidal ideation and means to carry out the plan Suicidal or homicidal gesture Overdose or other potentially serious attempt at self-harm Psychosis	**Do not delay treatment** Notify physician Multiple diagnostic studies or procedures Frequent consultation Continuous monitoring
Level 3: Moderate Risk	**Urgent**
Severe pain Suicidal/homicidal ideation with a plan and the means to carry out the plan Past inpatient psychiatric admission for depression Adolescent acting out, provocative or risk-taking behavior Recent childbirth, family loss, trauma, or emotional trauma Change in behavior, crying, or withdrawal Anxiety interferes with daily activity Signs of withdrawal, rapid heartbeat, diaphoresis, fever, auditory or visual hallucinations or delusions	**Refer for treatment as soon as possible** Monitor for changes in condition May need multiple diagnostic studies or procedures If abnormal vital signs, consider Level 2 Keep suicidal patient under observation while waiting to be seen Contact crisis or social worker, per facility protocol

(continued)

Level 4: Low Risk	Semi-Urgent
Moderate pain Suicidal thoughts without a plan or the means to carry out the plan Difficulty concentrating, sleeping, or maintaining interpersonal relationships Inability to experience pleasure Drug or alcohol ingestion or abuse Situational depression Change in medication or dose Out of medication History of eating disorder and postural vital signs	Reassess while waiting, per facility protocol Offer comfort measures May need a simple diagnostic study or procedure
Level 5: Lower Risk	Nonurgent
Reported history of depression with no current signs or symptoms History of posttraumatic stress disorder (PTSD)	Reassess while waiting, per facility protocol Offer comfort measures May need an examination only

RELATED PROTOCOLS:
Alcohol and Drug Use, Abuse, Overdose, and Dependence • Anxiety

NOTES

_____

_____

_____

_____

_____

_____

_____

_____

_____

_____

_____

_____

_____

_____

Diabetic Problems

KEY QUESTIONS:

Name • Age • Onset • Allergies • Prior History • Severity • Pain Scale • Vital Signs • Oxygen Saturation • Serum Glucose Level • Medications • Insulin Pump • Homecare Measures

ACUITY LEVEL/ASSESSMENT	NURSING CONSIDERATIONS
Level 1: Critical	**Resuscitation**
Apnea or severe respiratory distress Hypotension Unresponsive Pale, diaphoretic, and lightheaded or weak Seizure	**Refer for immediate treatment** Many resources needed Staff at bedside Mobilization of resuscitation team
Level 2: High Risk	**Emergent**
Altered mental status Intractable vomiting Blood glucose <60 mg/dL Hypoglycemic infant Insulin overdose Severe dehydration	**Do not delay treatment** Notify physician Multiple diagnostic studies or procedures Frequent consultation Constant monitoring Measure serum glucose level
Level 3: Moderate Risk	**Urgent**
Severe pain Blood glucose >400 mg/dL or <80 mg/dL Rapid respiratory rate Fruity breath odor Lightheaded Profuse diaphoresis Wound with signs of infection: drainage, fever, red streaks, or pus Persistent vomiting and inability to keep down medication Noncompliant with taking insulin or oral medication and feels ill	**Refer for treatment as soon as possible** May need multiple diagnostic studies or procedures Monitor for changes in condition If vital signs abnormal, consider Level 2 Measure serum glucose level

(continued)

Level 4: Low Risk	Semi-Urgent
Moderate pain Slow healing wound Upper respiratory infection with fever and cough Headache or nausea and prolonged period since last meal	Reassess while waiting, per facility protocol Offer comfort measures May need a simple diagnostic study or procedure
Level 5: Lower Risk	**Nonurgent**
Request for prescription refill New-onset insulin-dependent diabetes mellitus and requests additional education for self-administration of insulin	Reassess while waiting, per facility protocol Offer comfort measures May need examination only

RELATED PROTOCOLS:
Altered Mental Status • Fever • Wound Infection

NOTES

_____

_____

_____

_____

_____

_____

_____

_____

_____

_____

_____

_____

_____

_____

_____

_____

_____

_____

Diarrhea, Adult

KEY QUESTIONS:

Name • Age • Onset • Allergies • Prior History • Severity of Symptoms • Pain Scale • Vital Signs • Medications • Diet • Recent Travel • Other Family Members Ill • Laxatives • Chronic Diarrhea • Abdominal Surgery • Recent Antibiotic Therapy • Drinking From Wells or Streams

ACUITY LEVEL/ASSESSMENT	NURSING CONSIDERATIONS
Level 1: Critical	**Resuscitation**
Unresponsive Apnea or severe respiratory distress	**Refer for immediate treatment** Many resources needed Staff at bedside Mobilization of resuscitation team
Level 2: High Risk	**Emergent**
Confusion, lethargy, disorientation Altered mental status Severe weakness or lightheadedness Pallor, diaphoresis Large amounts of frank bloody stool At least two SIRS criteria: temperature >38.0°C or <36.0°C, HR >90, RR >20	**Do not delay treatment** Notify physician Multiple diagnostic studies or procedures Frequent consultation Continuous monitoring
Level 3: Moderate Risk	**Urgent**
Severe abdominal pain for longer than 2 hours Signs of dehydration: decreased urination, sunken eyes, loose dry skin, excessive thirst, dry mouth Lightheadedness upon standing Fever >101°F (38.3°C) and unresponsive to fever-reducing measures Diarrhea every 30–60 minutes for longer than 6 hours Diarrhea for more than 5 days Loss of bowel control Persistent vomiting for more than 3 days Recent international travel	**Refer for treatment as soon as possible** Monitor for changes in condition May need multiple diagnostic studies or procedures Collect/save stool specimen, per facility protocol If vital signs abnormal, consider Level 2 If tolerating oral fluids, give small amounts frequently

(continued)

Level 4: Low Risk	Semi-Urgent
Yellow, green, or frothy stool Moderate abdominal pain Diarrhea more than 6 times/24 hours Diarrhea for more than 2 days Low-grade fever Nausea	Reassess while waiting, per facility protocol Offer comfort measures May need simple diagnostic study or procedure
Level 5: Lower Risk	Nonurgent
Diarrhea more than 6 times/24 hours Loose stools	Reassess while waiting, per facility protocol Offer comfort measures May need examination only

RELATED PROTOCOLS:
Abdominal Pain, Adult • Poisoning, Exposure or Ingestion • Vomiting

NOTES
_____
_____
_____
_____
_____
_____
_____
_____
_____
_____
_____
_____
_____
_____
_____
_____

Diarrhea, Pediatric

KEY QUESTIONS:

Name • Age • Weight • Onset • Allergies • Prior History • Severity of Symptoms • Diaper Count • Pain Scale • Vital Signs • Medications • Diet • Recent Travel • Health of Family Members • Laxatives • Chronic Diarrhea • Abdominal Surgery • Recent Antibiotic Therapy • Drinking From Wells or Streams

ACUITY LEVEL/ASSESSMENT	NURSING CONSIDERATIONS
Level 1: Critical	**Resuscitation**
Unresponsive Apnea or severe respiratory distress Pale, diaphoretic, and lightheaded or weak Hypotensive	**Refer for immediate treatment** Many resources needed Staff at bedside Mobilization of resuscitation team
Level 2: High Risk	**Emergent**
Confusion, lethargy, disorientation Altered mental status Severe weakness or lightheadedness Cold, gray skin Large amounts of frank bloody stool Tachycardia Infant <12 weeks of age and fever >100.4°F (38.0°C) Capillary refill >2 seconds	**Do not delay treatment** Notify physician Multiple diagnostic studies or procedures Frequent consultation Constant monitoring
Level 3: Moderate Risk	**Urgent**
Signs of dehydration: age <1 year and no urine for more than 8 hours; age >1 year and no urine for more than 12 hours; sunken eyes or fontanels; crying without tears; excessive thirst; dry mouth Severe abdominal pain (drawing knees to chest with cramping)	**Refer for treatment as soon as possible** Reassess, per facility protocol Monitor for changes in condition May need multiple diagnostic studies or procedures Collect/save stool specimen, per facility protocol

(continued)

Level 3: Moderate Risk (*continued*)	Urgent
Lightheadedness upon standing Fever >105°F (40.6°C) and unresponsive to fever-reducing measures, >3 months old Age <1 month and diarrhea more than 3 times Age <1 year and diarrhea more than 8 times/8 hours Abdominal pain for more than 2 hours and no improvement with each episode of diarrhea Vomiting clear fluids and watery diarrhea more than 3 times Recent international travel	If vital signs abnormal, consider Level 2 If tolerating oral fluids, give small amounts frequently
Level 4: Low Risk	**Semi-Urgent**
Diarrhea for more than 3 days Fever unresponsive to fever-reducing measures Temperature >103°F (39.4°C) Temperature >101°F (38.3°C) for longer than 24 hours Bloody stools Receiving antibiotic therapy	Reassess while waiting, per facility protocol Offer comfort measures May need simple diagnostic study or procedure
Level 5: Lower Risk	**Nonurgent**
Chronic diarrhea Recent diet change Bloody stools and history of anal fissure	Reassess while waiting, per facility protocol Offer comfort measures May need examination only

RELATED PROTOCOLS:
Abdominal Pain, Pediatric • Poisoning, Exposure or Ingestion • Vomiting

NOTES

_____

_____

_____

_____

_____

_____

_____

Ear Problems

KEY QUESTIONS:

Name • Age • Onset • History • Temperature • Allergies • Medication • Pain Scale • Vital Signs

ACUITY LEVEL/ASSESSMENT	NURSING CONSIDERATIONS
Level 1: Critical	**Resuscitation**
Severe respiratory distress Pale, diaphoretic, and lightheaded or weak	**Refer for immediate treatment** Staff at bedside Mobilization of resuscitation team Many resources needed
Level 2: High Risk	**Emergent**
Confusion, lethargy, disorientation Altered mental status Injury and fluid leaking from ear Battle sign (bruising behind ear) with head trauma	**Do not delay treatment** Notify physician Multiple diagnostic studies or procedures Frequent consultation Continuous monitoring Check for CSF leakage with head trauma
Level 3: Moderate Risk	**Urgent**
Severe pain Pain, swelling, and bloody and/or purulent discharge from ear Redness or facial drooping on affected side of face associated with blow to head Sudden hearing loss with pain Pain unresponsive to analgesics History of diabetes/immunosuppression and ear pain	**Refer for treatment as soon as possible** Monitor for changes in condition May need multiple diagnostic studies or procedures If abnormal vital signs, consider Level 2

(continued)

Level 4: Low Risk	Semi-Urgent
Mild tenderness on bone behind ear Slight swelling, pain, warmth, drainage, low-grade fever Unable to remove wax plug with medication Decreased hearing, along with pain with cracking or popping noise Mild/intermittent ringing in ears Persistent earache after 3 days of antibiotics for ear infection	Reassess while waiting, per facility protocol Offer comfort measures May need a simple diagnostic study or procedure Do not instill liquid drops if eardrum rupture suspected
Level 5: Lower Risk	Nonurgent
Sunburn Itching Pain after exposure to cold Pain after swimming or exposure to water	Reassess while waiting, per facility protocol Offer comfort measures May need an examination only

RELATED PROTOCOLS:
Foreign Body, Ear

NOTES

_____

_____

_____

_____

_____

_____

_____

_____

_____

_____

_____

_____

_____

_____

Electric Shock/Lightning Injury

KEY QUESTIONS:

Name • Age • Onset • Cause • Vital Signs • Pain Scale • Entrance and Exit Wounds • Oxygen Saturation

ACUITY LEVEL/ASSESSMENT	NURSING CONSIDERATIONS
Level 1: Critical	**Resuscitation**
Apnea or severe respiratory distress Pulseless Unresponsive Pale, diaphoretic, and lightheaded or weak Hypotension	**Refer for immediate treatment** Staff at bedside Mobilization of resuscitation team Many resources needed
Level 2: High Risk	**Emergent**
Confusion, lethargy, disorientation Severe pain Altered mental status Weakness, chest pain, irregular pulse, palpitations Evidence of burn marks (entrance and/or exit wounds) Seizure Age <18 months History of unconsciousness Pallor, diaphoresis Oxygen saturation <92% on room air	**Do not delay treatment** Notify physician Multiple diagnostic studies or procedures Frequent consultation Continuous monitoring Monitor for internal injury, even if no external signs of burn are present Perform frequent extremity vascular checks Obtain 12-lead EKG as soon as possible Observe for entrance/exit burn wounds Start IV line if patient burned or monitoring shows abnormalities
Level 3: Moderate Risk	**Urgent**
History of cardiac disease Exposure to 220-W voltage or greater Burn to face Bloody/cloudy urine	**Refer for treatment as soon as possible** Monitor for changes in condition Monitor for internal injury, even with no external signs of burn

(*continued*)

Level 3: Moderate Risk (*continued*)	Urgent
Muscle pain Headache Fatigue	Perform frequent extremity vascular checks May need multiple diagnostic studies or procedures Obtain 12-lead EKG as soon as possible Apply dry dressing to burn wounds If abnormal vital signs, consider Level 2
Level 4: Low Risk	**Semi-Urgent**
Asymptomatic but parent or patient concerned	Reassess while waiting, per facility protocol Offer comfort measures May need simple diagnostic study or procedure

RELATED PROTOCOLS:
Chest Pain • Extremity Injury

NOTES

_____

_____

_____

_____

_____

_____

_____

_____

_____

_____

_____

_____

Extremity Injury

KEY QUESTIONS:

Name • Age • Onset • Allergies • Prior History • Severity • Pain Scale • Cause • Vital Signs • Oxygen Saturation • Neurovascular Status of Extremity

ACUITY LEVEL/ASSESSMENT	NURSING CONSIDERATIONS
Level 1: Critical	**Resuscitation**
Apnea or severe difficulty breathing Unresponsive Pulseless Pale, diaphoretic, and lightheaded or weak Pulsatile bleeding	**Refer for immediate treatment** Staff at bedside Mobilization of resuscitation team Many resources needed Apply pressure dressing to stop bleeding
Level 2: High Risk	**Emergent**
Altered mental status Severe pain in hip or thigh after traumatic injury and unable to ambulate Bone protrudes through the skin Partial or complete amputation Penetrating wound and object still present Unable to stop bleeding with pressure Fingers or toes of affected limb are cold, pale, mottled, or numb No pulse in affected extremity and cyanosis/pallor Prolonged capillary refill >2–3 seconds High-pressure injection injury	**Do not delay treatment** Notify physician Multiple diagnostic studies or procedures Frequent consultation Continuous monitoring Do not remove penetrating object Apply pressure dressing to stop bleeding
Level 3: Moderate Risk	**Urgent**
Deformed limb Severe pain with movement or weight-bearing Unable to move part of arm, hand, or foot distal to deep laceration	**Refer for treatment as soon as possible** May need multiple diagnostic studies or procedures Monitor for changes in condition

(continued)

Level 3: Moderate Risk (*continued*)	Urgent
Unable to remove ring and distal digit is turning pale, white, or blue Severe swelling, pain, and loss of sensation Increasing swelling or bruising around wound of person taking anticoagulants Puncture wound into a joint Numbness and tingling Open fracture Fever, drainage, red streaks	If vital signs abnormal, consider Level 2 Remove ring from swollen digit Apply splint, per facility protocol Elevate and apply ice pack for pain or swelling Assess ankle injury using Ottawa criteria Order radiographs, per facility protocol
Level 4: Low Risk	**Semi-Urgent**
Pain with movement or weight-bearing Difficulty moving the joint nearest the injury Puncture wound through sole of shoe Reported pop or snap at time of injury Suspicious history of injury (suspect abuse) Visible debris in wound after scrubbing History of diabetes No decrease in pain longer than 3 days after injury Numbness or tingling	Reassess while waiting, per facility protocol Offer comfort measures May need simple diagnostic study or procedure Remove ring from swollen digit Apply splint, per facility protocol Elevate and apply ice pack for pain or swelling Assess ankle injury using Ottawa criteria Order radiographs, per facility protocol
Level 5: Lower Risk	**Nonurgent**
Pain, swelling, or discoloration Chronic discomfort with old injury History of arthritis or tendonitis No reduction in swelling for more than 2 weeks after injury	Reassess while waiting, per facility protocol Offer comfort measures May need examination only

RELATED PROTOCOLS:
Electric Shock/Lightning Injury • Laceration • Puncture Wound

NOTES

_____

_____

_____

_____

_____

_____

Eye Injury or Problems

KEY QUESTIONS:

Name • Age • Onset • Cause • Allergies • Corrective Glasses or Contact Use • Visual Acuity • Vital Signs • Tetanus Immunization Status • Medications

ACUITY LEVEL/ASSESSMENT	NURSING CONSIDERATIONS
Level 1: Critical	**Resuscitation**
Apnea or severe respiratory distress Pulseless Unresponsive	**Refer for immediate treatment** Staff at bedside Mobilization of resuscitation team Many resources needed
Level 2: High Risk	**Emergent**
Altered mental status Laceration or penetrating injury to eye Blow or trauma to eye with marked loss of vision Flashing light in visual field Blood in iris (colored part of eye) Clear, jelly-like discharge from injured eye Corneal burn (exposure of eye to alkali or acid) Unilateral painless loss of vision	**Do not delay treatment** Notify physician Multiple diagnostic studies or procedures Frequent consultation Continuous monitoring Immediate irrigation for chemical burns Instill optic anesthetic, per facility protocol Consider C-spine injury with traumatic injury
Level 3: Moderate Risk	**Urgent**
Severe pain Burn to eye (thermal or light) Persistent blurred/double vision Swelling, pain, tearing of eye	**Refer for treatment as soon as possible** Monitor for changes in condition May need multiple diagnostic studies or procedures

(continued)

Level 3: Moderate Risk (*continued*)	Urgent
Eye pain associated with facial/orbital trauma Ecchymosis surrounding eye Increasing pain with eye movement Laceration to eyelid Foreign body in eye Recent eye surgery Swollen eyelids red, warm to touch, and fever >101.4°F (38.5°C)	Offer cool compresses to reduce swelling Instill optic anesthetic, per facility protocol If vital signs abnormal, consider Level 2
Level 4: Low Risk	**Semi-Urgent**
Discomfort or irritation persists 24 hours after injury or removal of foreign body Signs of infection develop after injury: mild pain, swelling, redness, drainage, or fever Small blood vessel rupture in sclera Fever <101.4°F (38.5°C) and swollen red eyelids or tear duct Persistent itching, redness, burning, and discharge History of improper contact lens usage, inability to remove contacts	Reassess while waiting, per facility protocol Offer comfort measures May need a simple diagnostic study or procedure For pepper spray or chili pepper exposure, may irrigate eye with whole milk (milk acts as a neutralizer)
Level 5: Lower Risk	**Nonurgent**
Dry eyes and itching Mild eye crusting Asymptomatic	Reassess while waiting, per facility protocol Offer comfort measures May need an examination only

RELATED PROTOCOLS:
Burns • Stroke

NOTES

_____

_____

_____

_____

_____

_____

Feeding Tube Problems

KEY QUESTIONS:

Name • Age • Prior History • Onset • Type of Tube • Length of Time Tube in Place • Pain Scale • Vital Signs

ACUITY LEVEL/ASSESSMENT	NURSING CONSIDERATIONS
Level 1: Critical	**Resuscitation**
Apnea or severe respiratory distress Unresponsive Pale, diaphoretic, and lightheaded or weak	**Refer for immediate treatment** Staff at bedside Mobilization of resuscitation team Many resources needed
Level 2: High Risk	**Emergent**
Altered mental status Severe bleeding through or at site of tube	**Do not delay treatment** Notify physician Multiple diagnostic studies or procedures Frequent consultation Continuous monitoring
Level 3: Moderate Risk	**Urgent**
Severe pain Swelling, bleeding, or foul-smelling purulent discharge at insertion site	**Refer for treatment as soon as possible** Monitor for change in condition May need multiple diagnostic studies or procedures If vital signs abnormal, consider Level 2
Level 4: Low Risk	**Semi-Urgent**
Moderate pain Signs of infection at insertion site: mild redness, swelling, pain, red streaks, or drainage Feeding tube dislodged or fallen out	Reassess while waiting, per facility protocol Offer comfort measures May need a simple diagnostic study or procedure

(continued)

Level 5: Lower Risk	Nonurgent
Tube frequently clogs after feeding or medication administration	Reassess while waiting, per facility protocol
Unable to unclog after trying home care measures	Offer comfort measures
Possible tube displacement	May need an examination only
Unable to pass solution into feeding tube	
Asymptomatic	

RELATED PROTOCOLS:
Abdominal Pain, Adult • Abdominal Pain, Pediatric • Wound Infection

NOTES

_____

_____

_____

_____

_____

_____

_____

_____

_____

_____

_____

_____

_____

_____

_____

_____

_____

_____

_____

_____

_____

Fever

KEY QUESTIONS:

Name • Age • Onset • Allergies • Medications • Prior History • Pain Scale • Vital Signs • Weight • Oxygen Saturation • Immunosuppressed • Recent Travel

ACUITY LEVEL/ASSESSMENT	NURSING CONSIDERATIONS
Level 1: Critical	**Resuscitation**
Apnea or severe respiratory distress Unresponsive Pale, diaphoretic, and lightheaded or weak	**Refer for immediate treatment** Staff at bedside Mobilization of resuscitation team Many resources needed
Level 2: High Risk	**Emergent**
Confusion or disorientation Altered mental status Excessive drooling or difficulty swallowing Age <12 weeks and temperature >100.4°F (38.0°C) Lethargy Petechiae Severe signs of dehydration or temperature >100.5°F (38.0°C) in elderly, pediatric, immunosuppressed, or otherwise compromised patient Anuria or decreased urine output for more than 24 hours Sunken eyes or fontanel, poor skin turgor, or excessive thirst in infant Severe headache, neck stiffness, neck pain, and photophobia At least two SIRS criteria: temperature >38.0°C or <36.0°C, HR >90, RR >20	**Do not delay treatment** Notify physician Multiple diagnostic studies or procedures Frequent consultation Continuous monitoring

(continued)

Level 3: Moderate Risk	Urgent

Severe pain
Temperature >104°F (40°C) and unresponsive to fever-reducing measures
Temperature >102°F (39°C) and
    Flank or back pain and painful/bloody urination
    Shortness of breath, pleuritic pain, wheezing and/or productive cough
    History of diabetes,
        cancer, HIV/AIDS, kidney/liver disease, pregnancy, or recent surgery
    Nausea/vomiting
Pediatric:
    Persistent irritability, inconsolable
    Infant age 3–6 months and rectal temperature >102°F (39°C) with diarrhea, vomiting, and dehydration
	Refer for treatment as soon as possible
	Monitor for change in condition
	May need multiple diagnostic studies or procedures
	If vital signs abnormal, consider Level 2
	Administer acetaminophen or ibuprofen, per facility protocol

Level 4: Low Risk	**Semi-Urgent**
Low-grade fever persists for more than 72 hours and no known cause Earache, sore throat, mildly swollen glands Rash Frequent urination and/or mild burning with urination Vaginal discharge	Reassess while waiting, per facility protocol Offer comfort measures May need a simple diagnostic study or procedure
Level 5: Lower Risk	**Nonurgent**
Temperature <101°F (38.2°C) with no other symptoms Recent immunization	Reassess while waiting, per facility protocol Offer comfort measures May need an examination only

RELATED PROTOCOLS:
Abdominal Pain, Adult • Abdominal Pain, Pediatric • Cold Symptoms •
Ear Problems • Sore Throat

NOTES

_____

_____

_____

_____

Finger and Toe Problems

KEY QUESTIONS:
Name • Age • Onset • Allergies • Prior History • Severity • Pain Scale • Vital Signs • Medications

ACUITY LEVEL/ASSESSMENT	NURSING CONSIDERATIONS
Level 1: Critical	**Resuscitation**
Apnea or severe respiratory distress Pulseless Unresponsive	**Refer for immediate treatment** Staff at bedside Mobilization of resuscitation team Many resources needed
Level 2: High Risk	**Emergent**
Altered mental status Open fracture Amputation Digits are cold, pale, blue, or mottled and numb	**Do not delay treatment** Notify physician Multiple diagnostic studies or procedures Frequent consultation Continuous monitoring
Level 3: Moderate Risk	**Urgent**
Severe pain Prolonged capillary refill Obvious deformity with compromised circulation Crush trauma Unable to stop bleeding with pressure Puncture wound into a joint Inability to remove rings, and digit is turning blue, pale, or white Fever, drainage, warm to touch, red streaks Exposed or injured nail bed Possible hair tourniquet in an infant and finger or toe swollen and discolored	**Refer for treatment as soon as possible** May need multiple diagnostic studies or procedures Monitor for change in condition Check capillary refill Monitor circulation, movement, and sensation of affected extremity If vital signs abnormal, consider Level 2 If possible, remove rings/jewelry before swelling worsens Do not remove penetrating object Apply pressure dressing to stop bleeding Apply splint, per facility protocol

(continued)

Level 4: Low Risk	Semi-Urgent
Moderate pain Swelling Decreased range of motion Bruising of the digit Subungual hematoma Pain and swelling at second metatarsophalangeal joint Numbness or tingling	Reassess while waiting, per facility protocol Offer comfort measures May need simple diagnostic study or procedure Elevate and apply ice pack for pain or swelling
Level 5: Lower Risk	Nonurgent
Pain or swelling without injury Minor bleeding under the nail Digit pain and history of arthritis or old injury	Reassess while waiting, per facility protocol Offer comfort measures May need examination only

RELATED PROTOCOLS:
Extremity Injury

NOTES

_____

_____

_____

_____

_____

_____

_____

_____

_____

_____

_____

_____

_____

_____

_____

_____

_____

Foreign Body, Ear

KEY QUESTIONS:

Name • Age • Onset • Identification of Foreign Body • Prior History • Medications • Allergies • Pain Scale • Vital Signs

ACUITY LEVEL/ASSESSMENT	NURSING CONSIDERATIONS
Level 1: Critical	**Resuscitation**
Severe respiratory distress Unresponsive Pale, diaphoretic, and lightheaded or weak	**Refer for immediate treatment** Staff at bedside Mobilization of resuscitation team Many resources needed
Level 2: High Risk	**Emergent**
Altered mental status Foreign body movement in ear causing hysteria (insect) Object impaled in ear CSF leaking from ear	**Do not delay treatment** Notify physician Multiple diagnostic studies or procedures Frequent consultation Continuous monitoring
Level 3: Moderate Risk	**Urgent**
Severe pain Unable to remove foreign body Facial drooping on side of injury Loss of coordination	**Refer for treatment as soon as possible** Monitor for change in condition May need multiple diagnostic studies or procedures If abnormal vital signs, consider Level 2
Level 4: Low Risk	**Semi-Urgent**
Foreign body in ear requiring simple removal Persistent discomfort Hearing loss Persistent bleeding for more than 30 minutes Lacerated earlobe Severe swelling of earlobe External ear red and swollen	Reassess while waiting, per facility protocol Offer comfort measures May need a simple diagnostic study or procedure

(continued)

Level 5: Lower Risk	Nonurgent
Foreign body removed but parent or patient concerned	Reassess while waiting, per facility protocol Offer comfort measures May need an examination only

RELATED PROTOCOLS:
Ear Problems • Laceration

NOTES

_____

_____

_____

_____

_____

_____

_____

_____

_____

_____

_____

_____

_____

_____

_____

_____

_____

_____

_____

_____

_____

_____

_____

Foreign Body, Ingested

KEY QUESTIONS:

Name • Age • Onset • Severity of Symptoms • Consideration for Poisoning • Foreign Object/Substance Ingested • Vital Signs • Medications

ACUITY LEVEL/ASSESSMENT	NURSING CONSIDERATIONS
Level 1: Critical	**Resuscitation**
Apnea or severe respiratory distress Pulseless Unresponsive	**Refer for immediate treatment** Staff at bedside Mobilization of resuscitation team Many resources needed
Level 2: High Risk	**Emergent**
Altered mental status Excessive salivation, drooling, or gagging Coughing, choking, or dyspnea Evidence of burn to lips and/or tongue Vomiting associated with possible corrosive substance Suicidal behavior Difficulty breathing Hematemesis Drooling Chest pain Poisonous substance	**Do not delay treatment** Notify physician Access Poison Control Center as necessary (1-800-222-1222) International Poison Control centers are also available Multiple diagnostic studies or procedures Frequent consultation Continual monitoring Observe suicidal patient until placed in a room
Level 3: Moderate Risk	**Urgent**
Severe pain Nausea and vomiting Object ingested larger than a nickel in children	**Refer for treatment as soon as possible** Engage family/emergency medical staff in identifying foreign object, if unknown

(*continued*)

Level 3: Moderate Risk (*continued*)	Urgent
Difficulty swallowing Sharp object or a button battery Abdominal distention Object ingested larger than a quarter in adult	Instruct parent/patient to check stool for object May need multiple diagnostic studies or procedures Monitor for change in condition If vital signs abnormal, consider Level 2 Access web-based Poison Control: www.webpoisoncontrol.org
Level 4: Low Risk	**Semi-Urgent**
Moderate pain Suspicious history or foreign body sensation	Reassess while waiting, per facility protocol Offer comfort measures May need simple diagnostic study or procedure
Level 5: Lower Risk	**Nonurgent**
Small wooden or plastic object or dull glass Object ingested smaller than a penny Asymptomatic but parent/patient is concerned	Reassess while waiting, per facility protocol Offer comfort measures May need examination only

RELATED PROTOCOLS:
Abdominal Pain, Adult • Abdominal Pain, Pediatric • Foreign Body, Inhaled

NOTES
_____
_____
_____
_____
_____
_____
_____
_____
_____
_____
_____
_____

Foreign Body, Inhaled

KEY QUESTIONS:

Name • Age • Onset • Allergies • Prior History • Severity of Symptoms • Pain Scale • Object Inhaled • Medications • Oxygen Saturation • Vital Signs

ACUITY LEVEL/ASSESSMENT	NURSING CONSIDERATIONS
Level 1: Critical	**Resuscitation**
Cyanosis Unresponsive Unable to speak Oxygen saturation <90% with oxygen Pulseless Choking	**Refer for immediate treatment** Staff at bedside Mobilization of resuscitation team Many resources needed
Level 2: High Risk	**Emergent**
Altered mental status Difficulty breathing Inspiratory stridor Bilateral wheezing Significant coughing Drooling Retractions Speaking in short sentences Oxygen saturation <90% on room air Oxygen saturation <94% with oxygen Pallor and diaphoresis Unequal breath sounds	**Do not delay treatment** Notify physician Multiple diagnostic studies or procedures Frequent consultation Continuous monitoring
Level 3: Moderate Risk	**Urgent**
Fever Severe pain Lightheadedness	**Refer for treatment as soon as possible** Monitor for change in condition

(continued)

Level 3: Moderate Risk (*continued*)	Urgent
Unilateral wheezing Expiratory wheezing Nasal flaring Speaking in partial sentences	May need multiple diagnostic studies or procedures If abnormal vital signs, consider Level 2
Level 4: Low Risk	**Semi-Urgent**
Sensation of foreign body with no respiratory signs and symptoms Speaking in full sentences	Reassess while waiting, per facility protocol Offer comfort measures May need a simple diagnostic study or procedure
Level 5: Lower Risk	**Nonurgent**
No symptoms but parent or patient concerned Oxygen saturation >95% on room air	Reassess while waiting, per facility protocol Offer comfort measures May need an examination only

RELATED PROTOCOLS:
Asthma • Breathing Problems • Foreign Body, Ingested

NOTES

_____

_____

_____

_____

_____

_____

_____

_____

_____

_____

_____

_____

_____

_____

Foreign Body, Inhaled

Foreign Body, Rectum or Vagina

KEY QUESTIONS:

Name • Age • Onset • Allergies • Prior History • Severity of Symptoms • Pain Scale • Vital Signs • Description of Object • Medications • Gender Identification

ACUITY LEVEL/ASSESSMENT	NURSING CONSIDERATIONS
Level 1: Critical	**Resuscitation**
Unresponsive Pale, diaphoretic, and confused or weak Violent assault with weapon (e.g., knife, blunt object) Severe respiratory distress	**Refer for immediate treatment** Many resources needed Staff at bedside Mobilization of resuscitation team
Level 2: High Risk	**Emergent**
Heavy rectal/vaginal bleeding Fever and systolic BP <100 mmHg Multiple injuries from assault Severe abdominal pain Altered mental status Traumatic injury to rectum or vagina with foreign object	**Do not delay treatment** Notify physician Multiple diagnostic studies or procedures Frequent consultation Constant monitoring
Level 3: Moderate Risk	**Urgent**
Urinary retention or hematuria Moderate rectal/vaginal bleeding Unable to remove foreign body High fever, chills, nausea, or vomiting Abdominal pain with movement Suspect sexual abuse Insertion of a sharp object	**Refer for treatment as soon as possible** Monitor for change in condition May need multiple diagnostic studies or procedures If vital signs abnormal, consider Level 2 If sexual abuse suspected and perpetrator present, move up to Level 2

(continued)

Level 4: Low Risk	Semi-Urgent
Sensation of rectal or vaginal fullness Rectal/vaginal pain Perirectal abscess Retained tampon or condom Scant rectal or vaginal bleeding Unable to pass stool	Reassess while waiting, per facility protocol Offer comfort measures May need simple diagnostic study or procedure
Level 5: Lower Risk	Nonurgent
Report of possible foreign body and no signs or symptoms	Reassess while waiting, per facility protocol Offer comfort measures May need examination only

RELATED PROTOCOLS:
Rectal Problems • Sexual Assault • Vaginal Bleeding, Abnormal

NOTES

_____

_____

_____

_____

_____

_____

_____

_____

_____

_____

_____

_____

_____

_____

_____

_____

_____

_____

Foreign Body, Skin

KEY QUESTIONS:

Name • Age • Onset • Allergies • Medications • Prior History • Severity • Pain Scale • Vital Signs • Tetanus Status

ACUITY LEVEL/ASSESSMENT	NURSING CONSIDERATIONS
Level 1: Critical	**Resuscitation**
Unresponsive Apnea or severe respiratory distress Pale, diaphoretic, and confused or weak	**Refer for immediate treatment** Staff at bedside Mobilization of resuscitation team Many resources needed
Level 2: High Risk	**Emergent**
Febrile and abnormal vital signs (BP <100 mmHg systolic) Fish hook imbedded in the eye Heavy bleeding from injury site Altered mental status Object impaled and difficulty breathing	**Do not delay treatment** Notify physician Multiple diagnostic studies or procedures Frequent consultation Continuous monitoring
Level 3: Moderate Risk	**Urgent**
Object impaled in the face and no respiratory impairment Severe pain Object imbedded in a joint space Object deeply imbedded Obvious injury to tendons, nerves, or vessels High level of anxiety Substance adhered to facial area (e.g., eyelids)	**Refer for treatment as soon as possible** May need multiple diagnostic studies or procedures Monitor for change in condition Obtain radiograph(s) for metal foreign body, per facility protocol Do not soak area of foreign body If abnormal vital signs, consider Level 2

(continued)

Level 4: Low Risk	Semi-Urgent
Nonremovable fish hook Object imbedded with minimal bleeding or no loss of sensation or function Moderate pain Foreign substance adhered to skin (e.g., tar, super glue) Signs of infection: redness, fever, pain, red streaks, warmth, pus	Reassess while waiting, per facility protocol Offer comfort measures May need simple diagnostic study or procedure
Level 5: Lower Risk	Nonurgent
Minimal pain Pierced earring inside an earlobe or other nonvital structure No symptoms but parent or patient concerned	Reassess while waiting, per facility protocol Offer comfort measures May need examination only

RELATED PROTOCOLS:
Laceration • Wound Infection

NOTES

_____

_____

_____

_____

_____

_____

_____

_____

_____

_____

_____

_____

_____

Genital Problems, Female

Name • Age • Onset • Allergies • Prior History • Severity • Pain Scale • Vital Signs • Medications • Gender Identification

ACUITY LEVEL/ASSESSMENT	NURSING CONSIDERATIONS
Level 1: Critical	**Resuscitation**
Severe respiratory distress Pale, diaphoretic, and lightheaded or weak Hypotension Unresponsive	**Refer for immediate treatment** Staff at bedside Mobilization of resuscitation team Many resources needed
Level 2: High Risk	**Emergent**
Altered mental status Trauma with heavy, pulsatile bleeding	**Do not delay treatment** Notify physician Multiple diagnostic studies or procedures Frequent consultation Continuous monitoring Do not remove penetrating object
Level 3: Moderate Risk	**Urgent**
History of genital surgery or mutilation and pain, bleeding, swelling, or drainage Severe pain Severe swelling of vulva Urinary retention Trauma to the area Vaginal prolapse Suspicion of human trafficking	**Refer for treatment as soon as possible** Monitor for change in condition May need multiple diagnostic studies or procedures If abnormal vital signs, consider Level 2

(continued)

Level 4: Low Risk	Semi-Urgent
Moderate vulvar pain Suspected sexually transmitted disease exposure Vaginal discharge, odor, itching Retained tampon, foreign object Vulvar swelling Fever and dysuria	Reassess while waiting, per facility protocol Offer comfort measures May need simple diagnostic study or procedure

RELATED PROTOCOLS:
Sexual Assault • Urination Problems

NOTES

_____

_____

_____

_____

_____

_____

_____

_____

_____

_____

_____

_____

_____

_____

_____

_____

_____

Genital Problems, Male

KEY QUESTIONS:

Name • Age • Onset • Allergies • Prior History • Severity • Pain Scale • Vital Signs • Medications • Gender Identification

ACUITY LEVEL/ASSESSMENT	NURSING CONSIDERATIONS
Level 1: Critical	**Resuscitation**
Severe respiratory distress Pale, diaphoretic, and lightheaded or weak Hypotension Unresponsive	**Refer for immediate treatment** Staff at bedside Mobilization of resuscitation team Many resources needed
Level 2: High Risk	**Emergent**
Altered mental status Trauma with heavy, pulsatile bleeding Sudden-onset unilateral testicular pain in patient <20 years of age Priapism Foreign body in penis	**Do not delay treatment** Notify physician Multiple diagnostic studies or procedures Frequent consultation Continuous monitoring Do not remove penetrating object
Level 3: Moderate Risk	**Urgent**
Blood at meatus Severe pain Fever and pain with urination Penis caught in zipper Severe swelling Urinary retention History of genital surgery Suspicion of human trafficking	**Refer for treatment as soon as possible** Monitor for change in condition May need multiple diagnostic studies or procedures If abnormal vital signs, consider Level 2

(*continued*)

Level 4: Low Risk	Semi-Urgent
Penile discharge with fever and pain Moderate pain Open sore or wound on penis Suspected sexually transmitted disease exposure Penile discharge Burning with urination	Reassess while waiting, per facility protocol Offer comfort measures May need simple diagnostic study or procedure
Level 5: Lower Risk	Nonurgent
Erectile dysfunction Pain during or after intercourse Loss of sexual interest	Reassess while waiting, per facility protocol Offer comfort measures May need an examination only

RELATED PROTOCOLS:
Urination Problems

NOTES

_____

_____

_____

_____

_____

_____

_____

_____

_____

_____

_____

_____

_____

_____

_____

Headache

KEY QUESTIONS:

Name • Age • Onset • Allergies • Medications • Prior History • Severity of Symptoms • Pain Scale • Vital Signs

ACUITY LEVEL/ASSESSMENT	NURSING CONSIDERATIONS
Level 1: Critical	**Resuscitation**
Apnea or severe respiratory distress Pale, diaphoretic, and lightheaded or weak Pulseless Hypotension Stroke signs and symptoms	**Refer for immediate treatment** Staff at bedside Mobilization of resuscitation team Many resources needed
Level 2: High Risk	**Emergent**
"Worst headache of my life" Fever and stiff or painful neck Sudden onset of unilateral weakness Altered mental status Difficulty speaking or swallowing Nuchal rigidity Hyperreflexia Facial droop Petechiae	**Do not delay treatment** Notify physician Multiple diagnostic studies or procedures Frequent consultation Continuous monitoring
Level 3: Moderate Risk	**Urgent**
Acute onset of severe headache Vomiting/nausea Vision changes Exposure to chemicals or smoke Recent head injury/trauma Known exposure to meningitis (bacterial)	**Refer for treatment as soon as possible** Monitor for change in condition May need multiple diagnostic studies or procedures If vital signs abnormal, consider Level 2

(continued)

Level 4: Low Risk	Semi-Urgent
Low-grade fever History of migraines and photosensitivity Body aches Acute stress Fever	Reassess while waiting, per facility protocol Offer comfort measures May need a simple diagnostic study or procedure
Level 5: Lower Risk	**Nonurgent**
Sinus symptoms Cold symptoms Caffeine withdrawal Pain occurs with reading No other symptoms but parent or patient concerned	Reassess while waiting, per facility protocol Offer comfort measures May need an examination only

RELATED PROTOCOLS:
Cold Symptoms • Fever • Head Injury
See Appendix K: Headache: Common Characteristics

NOTES

_____

_____

_____

_____

_____

_____

_____

_____

_____

_____

_____

_____

_____

_____

_____

_____

Head Injury

KEY QUESTIONS:

Name • Age • Onset • Allergies • Prior History • Severity of Symptoms • Pain Scale •
Vital Signs • Oxygen Saturation • Medications • Glasgow Coma Scale Score •
Concussion Protocol • Mechanism of Injury

ACUITY LEVEL/ASSESSMENT	NURSING CONSIDERATIONS
Level 1: Critical	**Resuscitation**
Unresponsive Seizure Apnea or severe respiratory distress Pale, diaphoretic, and lightheaded or weak Pulseless	**Refer for immediate treatment** Staff at bedside Mobilization of resuscitation team Many resources needed
Level 2: High Risk	**Emergent**
Altered mental status Severe neck pain Uncontrolled bleeding High-risk mechanism of injury Clear drainage from nose or ears Change in speech New-onset weakness or numbness Battle sign or raccoon eyes Obvious dent to head	**Do not delay treatment** Notify physician Multiple diagnostic studies or procedures Frequent consultation Continuous monitoring Protect C-spine Refer to MVA Triage Questions (Appendix L: MVA Triage Questions)
Level 3: Moderate Risk	**Urgent**
History of loss of consciousness, fine now Visual changes Vomiting more than three times or projectile vomiting	**Refer for treatment as soon as possible** Monitor for changes in condition May need multiple diagnostic studies or procedures If vital signs abnormal, consider Level 2

(continued)

Level 3: Moderate Risk (*continued*)	Urgent
Deceleration injury Infant fall >2 feet Suspect child abuse or neglect Loss of memory, fine now Change in balance or equilibrium Facial lacerations	Refer to Mechanisms of Injury (Appendices M: Mechanisms of Injury: Adult; N: Mechanisms of Injury: School Age and Adolescent [7–17 years old]; O: Mechanisms of Injury: Toddler and Preschooler [1–6 years old]; P: Mechanisms of Injury: Infant [birth to 1 year old]) Ice pack to help reduce swelling
Level 4: Low Risk	**Semi-Urgent**
Nausea Infant fall <2 feet Injury and no loss of consciousness Headache longer than 1 week post injury	Reassess while waiting, per facility protocol Offer comfort measures May need a simple diagnostic study or procedure
Level 5: Lower Risk	**Nonurgent**
No symptoms but parent or patient concerned	Reassess while waiting, per facility protocol Offer comfort measures May need an examination only

RELATED PROTOCOLS:

Headache • Traumatic Injury

See Appendices L: MVA Triage Questions; M: Mechanisms of Injury: Adult; N: Mechanisms of Injury: School Age and Adolescent (7–17 years old); O: Mechanisms of Injury: Toddler and Preschooler (1–6 years old); P: Mechanisms of Injury: Infant (birth to 1 year old)

NOTES

_____

_____

_____

_____

_____

_____

_____

_____

_____

Heart Rate, Rapid

KEY QUESTIONS:

Name • Age • Onset • Allergies • Medications • Prior History • Severity of Symptoms • Pain Scale • Vital Signs • Oxygen Saturation • Cardiac History (Stent, Coronary Artery Bypass Graft [CABG], Valve Replacement, Myocardial Infarction, Pacemakers, Automatic Implantable Cardioverter-Defibrillator [AICD], Implanted Device in Chest)

ACUITY LEVEL/ASSESSMENT	NURSING CONSIDERATIONS
Level 1: Critical	**Resuscitation**
Apnea or severe respiratory distress Unresponsive Pale, diaphoretic, and lightheaded or weak Hypotension	**Refer for immediate treatment** Many resources needed Staff at bedside Mobilization of resuscitation team
Level 2: High Risk	**Emergent**
Altered mental status Chest, jaw, or arm pain Adult HR >150 bpm Child HR >180 bpm Difficulty breathing Facial cyanosis or pallor Possible overdose Lightheadedness or dizziness Unsteady walking Diaphoresis Drug overdose Internal defibrillator in chest and repeated shocks	**Do not delay treatment** Notify physician Multiple diagnostic studies or procedures Frequent consultation Continuous monitoring
Level 3: Moderate Risk	**Urgent**

History of heart disease, paroxysmal supraven-
   tricular tachycardia, or thyroid disease
Intermittent episodes of fast heart rate
	Refer for treatment as soon as possible
	May need multiple diagnostic studies or
	   procedures

(continued)

Level 3: Moderate Risk (*continued*)	Urgent
History of antihistamine or diet pill use Signs of dehydration Possible drug ingestion or exposure Anxiety attack	Monitor for change in condition If vital signs abnormal, consider Level 2
Level 4: Low Risk	**Semi-Urgent**
Diarrhea Vomiting New medication Increased caffeine consumption Increased stress or emotional anxiety HR <140 bpm and regular	Reassess while waiting, per facility protocol Offer comfort measures May need a simple diagnostic study or procedure
Level 5: Lower Risk	**Nonurgent**
History of palpitations No symptoms Mild fever Associated pain or anxiety	Reassess while waiting, per facility protocol Offer comfort measures May need examination only

RELATED PROTOCOLS:
Anxiety • Breathing Problems • Chest Pain • Diarrhea, Adult • Diarrhea, Pediatric •
Lightheadedness/Fainting • Vomiting

NOTES

_____

_____

_____

_____

_____

_____

_____

_____

_____

_____

Heart Rate, Slow

KEY QUESTIONS:

Name • Age • Onset • Allergies • Medications • Prior History • Severity of Symptoms • Pain Scale • Vital Signs • Oxygen Saturation • Cardiac History (Stent, Coronary Artery Bypass Graft [CABG], Pacemaker, Myocardial Infarction, Internal Defibrillator)

ACUITY LEVEL/ASSESSMENT	NURSING CONSIDERATIONS
Level 1: Critical	**Resuscitation**
Apnea or severe respiratory distress Pale, diaphoretic, and lightheaded or weak Oxygen saturation <90% with oxygen Unresponsive	**Refer for immediate treatment** Many resources needed Staff at bedside Mobilization of resuscitation team
Level 2: High Risk	**Emergent**
Altered mental status Chest, neck, arm, or jaw pain Difficulty breathing Facial cyanosis or pallor Possible overdose of beta-blockers, thyroid medications, digoxin, or tricyclic antidepressants Systolic BP <90 mmHg Dizziness or lightheadedness Unsteady ambulation Drug overdose Diaphoresis	**Do not delay treatment** Notify physician Multiple diagnostic studies or procedures Frequent consultation Constant monitoring
Level 3: Moderate Risk	**Urgent**
New medication Unexplained weight gain, fatigue, chronically feeling "cold"	**Refer for treatment as soon as possible** May need multiple diagnostic studies or procedures

(continued)

Level 3: Moderate Risk (*continued*)	Urgent
History of heart disease, heart block, or pacemaker malfunction Nausea/vomiting Irregular heart rate	Monitor for change in condition If vital signs abnormal, consider Level 2
Level 4: Low Risk	**Semi-Urgent**
HR usually slow Athletic conditioning Eating disorder, heart rate <60 bpm, and dizziness with standing	Reassess while waiting, per facility protocol Offer comfort measures May need a simple diagnostic study or procedure
Level 5: Lower Risk	**Nonurgent**
Asymptomatic but parent or patient concerned	Reassess while waiting, per facility protocol Offer comfort measures May need examination only

RELATED PROTOCOLS:
Breathing Problems • Chest Pain • Lightheadedness/Fainting

NOTES

_____

_____

_____

_____

_____

_____

_____

_____

_____

_____

_____

_____

_____

_____

Heat Exposure

KEY QUESTIONS:

Name • Age • Onset • Temperature • Cardiac History • Hypertension • Diabetes • Vital Signs •
Oxygen Saturation • Medications • Prior History

ACUITY LEVEL/ASSESSMENT	NURSING CONSIDERATIONS
Level 1: Critical	**Resuscitation**
Apnea or severe respiratory distress Pulseless Unresponsive	**Refer for immediate treatment** Staff at bedside Mobilization of resuscitation team Many resources needed
Level 2: High Risk	**Emergent**
Confusion, lethargy, disorientation Altered mental status Profuse sweating with rapid heart rate (heat exhaustion) Signs of cardiovascular collapse/shock ($\downarrow$ blood pressure, $\uparrow$ heart rate, $\uparrow$ respiratory rate) Skin hot and dry with no sweating (heatstroke) Seizures	**Do not delay treatment** Notify physician Multiple diagnostic studies or procedures Frequent consultation Continuous monitoring
Level 3: Moderate Risk	**Urgent**
Severe pain Muscle cramps or loss of coordination Vomiting Dark yellow or orange urine Dizziness, faintness, weakness Age <10 years old or >70 years old	**Refer for treatment as soon as possible** Monitor for changes in condition May need multiple diagnostic studies or procedures If alert, encourage cold liquid intake Do not give acetaminophen or aspirin to lower temperature Place patient in cool, shady area If abnormal vital signs, consider Level 2

(continued)

Level 4: Low Risk	Semi-Urgent
Headache Nausea Flushing	Reassess while waiting, per facility protocol Offer comfort measures May need simple diagnostic study or procedure
Level 5: Lower Risk	Nonurgent
Symptoms improved with intake of oral fluids Asymptomatic	Reassess while waiting, per facility protocol Offer comfort measures May need an examination only

RELATED PROTOCOLS:
Confusion • Fever • Sunburn • Weakness

NOTES

Hip Pain/Injury

Name • Age • Onset • Allergies • Medications • Prior History • Mechanism of Injury • Severity of Symptoms • Pain Scale

ACUITY LEVEL/ASSESSMENT	NURSING CONSIDERATIONS
Level 1: Critical	**Resuscitation**
Unresponsive Pulseless Apnea or severe respiratory distress	**Refer for immediate treatment** Many resources needed Staff at bedside Mobilization of resuscitation team
Level 2: High Risk	**Emergent**
Altered mental status Cold, blue or gray foot/toes on affected side External or internal rotation and decreased motion, sensation, or circulation distally	**Do not delay treatment** Notify physician Multiple diagnostic studies or procedures Frequent consultation Constant monitoring
Level 3: Moderate Risk	**Urgent**
History of injury or fall External rotation of foot Immobility or deformity Severe pain Shortened limb Injury and history of bleeding problems Ecchymosis	**Refer for treatment as soon as possible** May need multiple diagnostic studies or procedures Monitor for change in condition If vital signs abnormal, consider Level 2
Level 4: Low Risk	**Semi-Urgent**
Moderate pain with movement History of joint replacement or surgery	Reassess while waiting, per facility protocol Offer comfort measures May need a simple diagnostic study or procedure

(continued)

Level 5: Lower Risk	Nonurgent
Chronic hip or joint pain Pain increases with activity Pain relieved by OTC medications	Reassess while waiting, per facility protocol Offer comfort measures May need examination only

RELATED PROTOCOLS:
Extremity Injury • Traumatic Injury

NOTES

_____

_____

_____

_____

_____

_____

_____

_____

_____

_____

_____

_____

_____

_____

_____

_____

_____

_____

_____

_____

_____

_____

_____

_____

Hives

Name • Age • Onset • Allergies • Prior History • Severity of Symptoms • Pain Scale • Suspected Cause • Medications • Vital Signs • Recent Changes in Food or Medication • Recent Contrast Media

ACUITY LEVEL/ASSESSMENT	NURSING CONSIDERATIONS
Level 1: Critical	**Resuscitation**
Severe difficulty breathing Unresponsive Pale, diaphoretic, and lightheaded or weak Unable to speak Severe swelling of tongue or throat	**Refer for immediate treatment** Staff at bedside Mobilization of resuscitation team Many resources needed
Level 2: High Risk	**Emergent**

Altered mental status
Prior anaphylaxis requiring epinephrine
Urticaria and hives throughout body
Speaking in short sentences
Hives and rapidly progressing:
    Drooling
    Difficulty swallowing
    Difficulty breathing
    Wheezing
    Chest tightness
    Swelling of tongue or throat
	Do not delay treatment
	Notify physician
	Multiple diagnostic studies or procedures
	Frequent consultation
	Continuous monitoring

Level 3: Moderate Risk	**Urgent**
Nausea or vomiting Abdominal pain/diarrhea Severe pain or distress Lightheadedness Facial or lip swelling Inability to speak in full sentences Contact with known allergen	**Refer for treatment as soon as possible** Monitor for change in condition May need a breathing treatment while waiting, per facility protocol May need multiple diagnostic studies or procedures If vital signs abnormal, consider Level 2

Level 4: Low Risk	Semi-Urgent
Swelling of extremities Diarrhea Speaking in full sentences Hives respond to antihistamines New onset with emotional stimulus Moderate discomfort	Reassess while waiting, per facility protocol Offer comfort measures May need a simple diagnostic study or procedure
Level 5: Lower Risk	Nonurgent
History of a viral illness Hives have resolved	Reassess while waiting, per facility protocol Offer comfort measures May need an examination only

RELATED PROTOCOLS:
Allergic Reaction • Bee Sting • Breathing Problems • Rash, Adult and Pediatric

NOTES

_____

_____

_____

_____

_____

_____

_____

_____

_____

_____

_____

_____

_____

_____

_____

_____

_____

_____

_____

Hypertension

KEY QUESTIONS:

Name • Age • Onset • Allergies • Prior History • Medications • Severity • Pain Scale • Associated Symptoms • Vital Signs • Oxygen Saturation • Last Elevated Blood Pressure Reading

ACUITY LEVEL/ASSESSMENT	NURSING CONSIDERATIONS
Level 1: Critical	**Resuscitation**
Apnea or severe respiratory distress Unresponsive Pulseless Pale, diaphoretic, and lightheaded or weak	**Refer for immediate treatment** Staff at bedside Mobilization of resuscitation team Many resources needed
Level 2: High Risk	**Emergent**
Altered mental status Severe weakness History of thoracic or abdominal dissection Persistent numbness and tingling in hands and feet Coughing up blood or blood-tinged sputum Difficulty breathing Persistent nosebleed Diastolic BP >110 mmHg Systolic BP >180 mmHg Severe headache, blurred vision, nausea, or vomiting Chest, neck, shoulders, jaw, or back pain	**Refer for treatment within minutes** Notify physician Administer oxygen per facility protocol Perform 12-lead EKG per facility protocol Provide IV access per facility protocol Many diagnostic studies or procedures Frequent consultation Continuous monitoring
Level 3: Moderate Risk	**Urgent**
History of heart disease, diabetes, congestive heart failure, clotting disorders, sleep apnea, kidney problems, adrenal gland tumor, thyroid problems Use of recreational drugs	**Refer for treatment as soon as possible** Monitor for changes in condition May need multiple diagnostic studies or procedures If abnormal vital signs, consider Level 2 Consider 12-lead EKG per facility protocol

(continued)

Level 4: Low Risk	Semi-Urgent
Periods of dizziness after starting new blood pressure medication Receiving treatment for hypertension and persistent blood pressure >160/100 mmHg Intermittent nosebleed Strong family history of heart disease, heart attack, stroke, or diabetes	Reassess while waiting, per facility protocol Offer comfort measures May need simple diagnostic study or procedure
Level 5: Lower Risk	Nonurgent
Persistent BP readings >140/90 mmHg	Reassess while waiting, per facility protocol Offer comfort measures May need examination only

RELATED PROTOCOLS:
Breathing Problems • Chest Pain • Heart Rate, Rapid • Heart Rate, Slow

NOTES

_____

_____

_____

_____

_____

_____

_____

_____

_____

_____

_____

_____

_____

_____

_____

_____

_____

Itching Without a Rash

KEY QUESTIONS:
Name • Age • Onset • Allergies • Medications • Prior History • Severity of Symptoms • Pain Scale • Vital Signs

ACUITY LEVEL/ASSESSMENT	NURSING CONSIDERATIONS
Level 1: Critical	**Resuscitation**
Severe respiratory distress Hypotension Unresponsive	**Refer for immediate treatment** Many resources needed Staff at bedside Mobilization of resuscitation team
Level 2: High Risk	**Emergent**
Altered mental status	**Do not delay treatment** Notify physician Multiple diagnostic studies or procedures Frequent consultation Constant monitoring
Level 3: Moderate Risk	**Urgent**
Itching started after taking new medication Severe pain Onset occurred after exposure to a known allergen Recent drug withdrawal	**Refer for treatment as soon as possible** May need multiple diagnostic studies or procedures Monitor for change in condition If vital signs abnormal, consider Level 2
Level 4: Low Risk	**Semi-Urgent**
Jaundiced skin Persistent itching Open wounds from scratching Vaginal itching	Reassess while waiting, per facility protocol Offer comfort measures May need a simple diagnostic study or procedure

(continued)

Level 5: Lower Risk	Nonurgent
Generalized itching Itching around genitals Lice, crabs, or nits present Contact dermatitis Exposure to poison ivy or poison oak Rectal itching	Reassess while waiting, per facility protocol Offer comfort measures May need examination only

RELATED PROTOCOLS:
Jaundice • Rectal Problems

NOTES

_____

_____

_____

_____

_____

_____

_____

_____

_____

_____

_____

_____

_____

_____

_____

_____

_____

_____

_____

_____

_____

_____

Jaundice

Name • Age • Onset • Allergies • Prior History • Medications • Pain Scale • Vital Signs

ACUITY LEVEL/ASSESSMENT	NURSING CONSIDERATIONS
Level 1: Critical	**Resuscitation**
Severe difficulty breathing Pale, diaphoretic, and lightheaded or weak Unresponsive	**Refer for immediate treatment** Many resources needed Staff at bedside Mobilization of resuscitation team
Level 2: High Risk	**Emergent**
Altered mental status	**Do not delay treatment** Notify physician Multiple diagnostic studies or procedures Frequent consultation Continuous monitoring
Level 3: Moderate Risk	**Urgent**
Malnutrition and weight loss Signs of dehydration Fever Immunosuppressed, diabetic, or pregnant Severe pain Liver transplant	**Refer for treatment as soon as possible** Monitor for changes in condition May need multiple diagnostic studies or procedures If abnormal vital signs, consider Level 2
Level 4: Low Risk	**Semi-Urgent**

Known or suspected exposure to blood-borne
   pathogens
Dark urine
Clay-colored stools
	Reassess while waiting, per facility protocol
	Offer comfort measures
	May need a simple diagnostic study or
	   procedure

(continued)

Level 4: Low Risk (*continued*)	Semi-Urgent
Vomiting Abdominal pain Loss of appetite Age <10 years old or >70 years old New onset but no other symptoms Known liver disease	
Level 5: Lower Risk	**Nonurgent**
Prior history of jaundice and no other symptoms	Reassess while waiting, per facility protocol Offer comfort measures May need an examination only

RELATED PROTOCOLS:
Abdominal Pain, Adult • Fever • Itching Without a Rash

NOTES

_____

_____

_____

_____

_____

_____

_____

_____

_____

_____

_____

_____

_____

_____

_____

_____

_____

_____

Jaundice, Newborn

KEY QUESTIONS:
Name • Age • Onset • Allergies • Prior History • Medications • Vital Signs • Birth History

ACUITY LEVEL/ASSESSMENT	NURSING CONSIDERATIONS
Level 1: Critical	**Resuscitation**
Apnea or severe respiratory distress Unresponsive Pale and weak or not moving	**Refer for immediate treatment** Many resources needed Staff at bedside Mobilization of resuscitation team
Level 2: High Risk	**Emergent**
Altered mental status Jaundice below the waistline	**Do not delay treatment** Notify physician Multiple diagnostic studies or procedures Frequent consultation Continuous monitoring
Level 3: Moderate Risk	**Urgent**
No wet diapers for more than 8 hours Decreased oral intake Decreased activity Signs of dehydration: poor skin turgor, sunken eyes or fontanel, crying without tears Fever >100.4°F (38.0°C) Temperature <96.8°F (36.0°C) Jaundice in newborn within first 24 hours of life Family history of Gilbert's syndrome, liver disease, or hemolytic disorders	**Refer for treatment as soon as possible** Monitor for changes in condition May need multiple diagnostic studies or procedures If abnormal vital signs, consider Level 2

(continued)

Level 4: Low Risk	Semi-Urgent
Worsening jaundice for more than 7 days No stool for more than 24 hours Stools white, yellow, or gray	Reassess while waiting, per facility protocol Offer comfort measures May need a simple diagnostic study or procedure
Level 5: Lower Risk	Nonurgent
No other symptoms but parents concerned Onset of jaundice after 7 days of age	Reassess while waiting, per facility protocol Offer comfort measures May need an examination only

RELATED PROTOCOLS:
Abdominal Pain, Pediatric • Crying Baby • Fever • Rash, Adult and Pediatric

NOTES

Knee Pain and/or Swelling

KEY QUESTIONS:

Name • Age • Onset • Allergies • Medications • Prior History • Pain Scale • Vital Signs • Traumatic Injury

ACUITY LEVEL/ASSESSMENT	NURSING CONSIDERATIONS
Level 1: Critical	**Resuscitation**
Apnea or severe respiratory distress Unresponsive Pale, diaphoretic, and lightheaded or weak Pulseless	**Refer for immediate treatment** Staff at bedside Mobilization of resuscitation team Many resources needed
Level 2: High Risk	**Emergent**
Altered mental status Cyanosis of foot or leg on affected side Chest pain Difficulty breathing Pale, paralyzed, or markedly weak leg Obvious deformity Knee dislocation (orthopedic emergency)	**Do not delay treatment** Notify physician Multiple diagnostic studies or procedures Frequent consultation Continuous monitoring
Level 3: Moderate Risk	**Urgent**
Severe pain History of acute trauma Leg numb	**Refer for treatment as soon as possible** May need multiple diagnostic studies or procedures Monitor for change in condition Offer wheelchair and elevate extremity Offer ice pack for known injury If vital signs abnormal, consider Level 2

(continued)

Level 4: Low Risk	Semi-Urgent
Moderate pain Inability to bear weight Red, swollen, hot joint Pain and swelling increasing with activity Knee locking or popping Recent knee surgery	Reassess while waiting, per facility protocol Offer comfort measures May need simple diagnostic study or procedure
Level 5: Lower Risk	Nonurgent
Chronic or intermittent pain or swelling Knee buckling or locking	Reassess while waiting, per facility protocol Offer comfort measures May need examination only

RELATED PROTOCOLS:
Extremity Injury • Traumatic Injury

NOTES

_____

_____

_____

_____

_____

_____

_____

_____

_____

_____

_____

_____

_____

_____

_____

_____

_____

Laceration

KEY QUESTIONS:

Name • Age • Onset • Allergies • Medications • Prior History • Mechanism of Injury • Severity • Pain Scale • Vital Signs • Last Tetanus Immunization

ACUITY LEVEL/ASSESSMENT	NURSING CONSIDERATIONS
Level 1: Critical	**Resuscitation**
Apnea or severe respiratory distress Pulseless Unresponsive Pale, diaphoretic, and lightheaded or weak	**Refer for immediate treatment** Staff at bedside Mobilization of resuscitation team Many resources needed
Level 2: High Risk	**Emergent**
Altered mental status Pulsatile bleeding Exposure of deep structures (tissue, tendons, organs, bone, etc.) Laceration near a major artery No pulse distal to laceration Cyanotic distal to laceration Impaled object Gaping, bleeding wound	**Do not delay treatment** Notify physician Multiple diagnostic studies or procedures Frequent consultation Continuous monitoring Leave impaled object in place Apply compression dressing to control bleeding
Level 3: Moderate Risk	**Urgent**
Severe pain Gaping wound with bleeding controlled History of bleeding disorder Laceration involves a joint Decreased range of motion of the limb Facial laceration Contaminated wound	**Refer for treatment as soon as possible** Reassess while waiting, per facility protocol May need multiple diagnostic studies or procedures Monitor for changes in condition If vital signs abnormal, consider Level 2

(*continued*)

Level 4: Low Risk	Semi-Urgent
Moderate pain Taking anticoagulant (bleeding controlled) Signs of infection Road abrasions Stable laceration(s) with bleeding controlled, awaiting cleaning and suturing	Reassess while waiting, per facility protocol Offer comfort measures May need simple diagnostic study or procedure
Level 5: Lower Risk	**Nonurgent**
Minor laceration in need of cleaning and minimal repair	Reassess while waiting, per facility protocol Offer comfort measures May need examination only

RELATED PROTOCOLS:
Wound Infection

NOTES

_____

_____

_____

_____

_____

_____

_____

_____

_____

_____

_____

_____

_____

_____

_____

_____

_____

Lightheadedness/Fainting

KEY QUESTIONS:

Name • Age • Onset • Prior History • Fluid Intake • Medication • Pain Scale • Vital Signs • Oxygen Saturation

ACUITY LEVEL/ASSESSMENT	NURSING CONSIDERATIONS
Level 1: Critical	**Resuscitation**
Apnea or severe respiratory distress Pulseless Unresponsive Pale, diaphoretic, and lightheaded or weak	**Refer for immediate treatment** Staff at bedside Mobilization of resuscitation team Many resources needed
Level 2: High Risk	**Emergent**
Severe pain Confusion, lethargy, disorientation Altered mental status Weakness or inability to move arms or legs Difficulty speaking, disturbed vision Irregular heart rate or palpitations Chest pain	**Do not delay treatment** Notify physician Multiple diagnostic studies or procedures Frequent consultation Continuous monitoring
Level 3: Moderate Risk	**Urgent**
Recent head trauma with nausea or vomiting Moderate to severe vomiting or diarrhea Bleeding and tachycardia Postural vital signs Persistent headache or change in vision Diabetes	**Refer for treatment as soon as possible** Monitor for changes in condition May need multiple diagnostic studies or procedures Measure serum glucose level If abnormal vital signs, consider Level 2

(*continued*)

Level 4: Low Risk	Semi-Urgent
Symptoms interfere with activities Symptoms occur after taking new medication Symptoms occur with head movement Pregnancy or LMP >6 weeks Exposure to sun or hot environment Earache, tinnitus, loss of hearing	Reassess while waiting, per facility protocol Offer comfort measures May need a simple diagnostic study or procedure
Level 5: Lower Risk	**Nonurgent**
History of dieting Increased stress, emotional event, or hyperventilation Symptoms occur with alcohol consumption	Reassess while waiting, per facility protocol Offer comfort measures May need an examination only

RELATED PROTOCOLS:
Abdominal Pain, Adult • Abdominal Pain, Pediatric • Alcohol and Drug Use, Abuse, Overdose, and Dependence • Altered Mental Status • Chest Pain • Diarrhea, Adult • Diarrhea, Pediatric • Headache • Vaginal Bleeding, Abnormal • Vomiting

NOTES

_____

_____

_____

_____

_____

_____

_____

_____

_____

_____

_____

_____

_____

Menstrual Problems

KEY QUESTIONS:

Name • Age • Onset • Allergies • Medications • Prior History • Severity • Pain Scale • Vital Signs • Number of Saturated Pads or Tampons per Hour • Birth Control • Possibility of Pregnancy • Trauma

ACUITY LEVEL/ASSESSMENT	NURSING CONSIDERATIONS
Level 1: Critical	**Resuscitation**
Apnea or severe respiratory distress Unresponsive Pale, diaphoretic, and lightheaded or weak Pulseless	**Refer for immediate treatment** Staff at bedside Mobilization of resuscitation team Many resources needed
Level 2: High Risk	**Emergent**
Altered mental status Hypotensive Partial or complete expulsion of products of conception Persistent bleeding saturating more than two regular-size pads or tampons per hour for more than 2 hours Severe pain and possibility of pregnancy Sexually active, last period more than 6 weeks prior, and abdominal or shoulder pain Suspicion of human trafficking	**Do not delay treatment** Notify physician Multiple diagnostic studies or procedures Frequent consultation Continuous monitoring
Level 3: Moderate Risk	**Urgent**
Severe pain Heavy vaginal bleeding with clots Saturating one regular-size pad per hour for more than 6 hours Fainting or lightheadedness sitting or standing up Use of tampons and sudden high fever, sunburn-type rash, general ill feeling, lightheadedness, vomiting, watery diarrhea, tachycardia, or headache	**Refer for treatment as soon as possible** May need multiple diagnostic studies or procedures Monitor for changes in condition If vital signs abnormal, consider Level 2

(continued)

Level 4: Low Risk	Semi-Urgent
Cramping interferes with daily activity Persistent vaginal discharge Persistent vaginal bleeding for more than 10 days or less than 21 days since last period Possible pregnancy, bleeding, and no pain No menses and taking birth control pills	Reassess while waiting, per facility protocol Offer comfort measures May need simple diagnostic study or procedure
Level 5: Lower Risk	Nonurgent
Unusually heavy menstrual flow Scant menstruation Period missed or delayed and age >40 years	Reassess while waiting, per facility protocol Offer comfort measures May need examination only

RELATED PROTOCOLS:
Abdominal Pain, Adult • Vaginal Bleeding, Abnormal

NOTES

_____

_____

_____

_____

_____

_____

_____

_____

_____

_____

_____

_____

_____

_____

_____

_____

_____

Mouth Problems

KEY QUESTIONS:

Name • Age • Onset • Allergies • Medications • Prior History • Severity • Pain Scale • Vital Signs • Oxygen Saturation • Piercings • Recent Dental Work

ACUITY LEVEL/ASSESSMENT	NURSING CONSIDERATIONS
Level 1: Critical	**Resuscitation**
Apnea or severe respiratory distress Pulseless Unresponsive Sudden swelling in back of throat or tongue Injury impedes airway Pale, diaphoretic, and lightheaded or weak	**Refer for immediate treatment** Staff at bedside Mobilization of resuscitation team Many resources needed
Level 2: High Risk	**Emergent**
Altered mental status Inability to open/close mouth, jaw locked in place Penetrating injury to the back of the mouth Uncontrolled bleeding Traumatic injury that may potentially impede airway "Kissing tonsils" (unable to swallow own saliva) Drooling Tongue amputation	**Do not delay treatment** Notify physician Multiple diagnostic studies or procedures Frequent consultation Continuous monitoring Maintain airway
Level 3: Moderate Risk	**Urgent**
Severe pain not relieved with OTC medications or ice pack Gaping lacerations Facial swelling with unobstructed airway "Kissing tonsils" (unable to swallow own saliva) Difficulty speaking Use of bisphosphonates (risk of jaw osteonecrosis) Pain with facial swelling	**Refer for treatment as soon as possible** May need multiple diagnostic studies or procedures Monitor for change in condition Control bleeding If vital signs abnormal, consider Level 2

(continued)

Level 4: Low Risk	Semi-Urgent
Moderate pain Foul taste or odor from mouth Open sores, blisters, or white patches Fever and mouth sores	Reassess while waiting, per facility protocol Offer comfort measures May need simple diagnostic study or procedure
Level 5: Lower Risk	Nonurgent
Dental caries and pain Red or tender gums Sore spot on tongue	Reassess while waiting, per facility protocol Offer comfort measures May need examination only

RELATED PROTOCOLS:
Breathing Problems • Sore Throat • Toothache/Tooth Injury

NOTES

Neck Pain

KEY QUESTIONS:

Name • Age • Onset • Allergies • Medications • Prior History • Mechanism of Injury • Pain Scale • Vital Signs • Oxygen Saturation

ACUITY LEVEL/ASSESSMENT	NURSING CONSIDERATIONS
Level 1: Critical	**Resuscitation**
Apnea or severe respiratory distress Pulseless Unresponsive High-risk mechanism of injury with neurologic deficits Pale, diaphoretic, and lightheaded or weak	**Refer for immediate treatment** Staff at bedside Mobilization of resuscitation team Many resources needed
Level 2: High Risk	**Emergent**
Altered mental status High-risk mechanism of injury with no neurologic deficits Sudden onset of chest, jaw, or neck pain (no known injury) Difficulty breathing Severe headache and fever >101.3°F (38.5°C) Petechiae Sudden onset of numbness, tingling, weakness in both arms or legs Diaphoresis, palpitations, nausea, and/or vomiting Severe pain	**Do not delay treatment** Notify physician Multiple diagnostic studies or procedures Frequent consultation Continuous monitoring
Level 3: Moderate Risk	**Urgent**
Neck pain worsens with flexion Low-risk mechanism of injury Photophobia Nausea and vomiting Weakness or numbness in one arm	**Refer for treatment as soon as possible** May need multiple diagnostic studies or procedures Monitor for changes in condition If vital signs abnormal, consider Level 2

(continued)

Level 4: Low Risk	Semi-Urgent
Moderate neck pain worsens with extension Swollen glands, sore throat, cold symptoms, earache Swelling on one or both sides of neck Pain interferes with daily activity	Reassess while waiting, per facility protocol Offer comfort measures May need simple diagnostic study or procedure
Level 5: Lower Risk	Nonurgent
Neck pain without history of trauma or illness Chronic neck pain Slept in awkward position	Reassess while waiting, per facility protocol Offer comfort measures May need examination only

RELATED PROTOCOLS:
Chest Pain • Ear Problems • Fever • Head Injury • Sore Throat • Toothache/Tooth Injury

NOTES

_____

_____

_____

_____

_____

_____

_____

_____

_____

_____

_____

_____

_____

_____

_____

_____

Nosebleed

KEY QUESTIONS:
Name • Age • Onset • Allergies • Prior History • Medications • Pain Scale • Vital Signs • Oxygen Saturation • Immunocompromised

ACUITY LEVEL/ASSESSMENT	NURSING CONSIDERATIONS
Level 1: Critical	**Resuscitation**
Apnea or severe respiratory distress Pulseless Unresponsive Pale, diaphoretic, dizzy, or weak	**Refer for immediate treatment** Staff at bedside Mobilization of resuscitation team Many resources needed
Level 2: High Risk	**Emergent**
Altered mental status Abnormal vital signs Uncontrolled bleeding with clots Recent international travel (to a country with Ebola risk)	**Do not delay treatment** Notify physician Multiple diagnostic studies or procedures Frequent consultation Continuous monitoring Per facility protocol, provide IV access, draw laboratory samples, consider blood type and crossmatch
Level 3: Moderate Risk	**Urgent**
Severe pain Moderate to heavy bleeding (anterior bleed) Bleeding from nasal or facial trauma Hemoptysis Bleeding uncontrolled after 30 minutes of direct pressure	**Refer for treatment as soon as possible** May need multiple diagnostic studies or procedures Monitor for change in condition If abnormal vital signs, consider Level 2 Instruct patient to gently blow through the nose to clear nares

(continued)

Level 3: Moderate Risk (*continued*)	Urgent
History of bleeding disorder or other hematologic disease (leukemia, thrombocytopenia, etc.) and intermittent nosebleeds Headache Normal vital signs and lightheadedness Posterior nosebleed History of drug abuse, alcohol abuse, smoking, liver disease, or cancer	Administer nasal spray to help control bleeding, per facility protocol Clamp nose for 10 minutes
Level 4: Low Risk	**Semi-Urgent**
Intermittent nosebleed (more than three times in past 48 hours) Recent nasal surgery Frequent use of cocaine Moderate pain Foreign body in the nares	Reassess while waiting, per facility protocol Offer comfort measures May need a simple diagnostic study or procedure
Level 5: Lower Risk	**Nonurgent**
Seasonal allergies Frequent use of nasal sprays History of frequent controlled nosebleeds	Reassess while waiting, per facility protocol Offer comfort measures May need an examination only

RELATED PROTOCOLS:
Cold Symptoms • Foreign Body, Inhaled

NOTES

_____

_____

_____

_____

_____

_____

_____

_____

_____

_____

Poisoning, Exposure or Ingestion

KEY QUESTIONS:

Name • Age • Weight • Onset • Amount • Emesis After Ingestion • Allergies • Prior History • Medications • Pain Scale • Vital Signs • Oxygen Saturation • Name of Agent (If Known)

ACUITY LEVEL/ASSESSMENT	NURSING CONSIDERATIONS
Level 1: Critical	**Resuscitation**
Apnea or severe respiratory distress Pulseless Unresponsive Status epilepticus	**Refer for immediate treatment** Staff at bedside Mobilization of resuscitation team Many resources needed Contact National Poison Control Center for advice (1-800-222-1222)
Level 2: High Risk	**Emergent**
Altered mental status Lethargy Chest pain Recent seizure or postictal Wheezing, stridor, shortness of breath Ingestion of an acid, alkali, or hydrocarbon agent Burns on lips or tongue Cyanosis Unstable vital signs Suicide attempt Constricted or dilated pupils Known carbon monoxide exposure Strong suspicion of exposure to chemical agent and symptomatic Excessive drooling, sweating, or hyperactive reflexes Fever >104°F (40.0°C) Child found with open medication bottle or other potentially dangerous substances	**Do not delay treatment** Notify physician Multiple diagnostic studies or procedures Frequent consultation Continuous monitoring Contact National Poison Control Center for advice (1-800-222-1222) Provide IV access, perform 12-lead EKG, per facility protocol If suicide attempt, place in observed area until bed available If multiple patients with similar symptoms, consider chemical exposure and initiate decontamination procedures per facility plan

(continued)

Level 3: Moderate Risk	Urgent
Severe pain Nausea, vomiting, diarrhea Abdominal pain Headache Ataxia Dizziness or lightheadedness Psychiatric history Cognitive dysfunction Irritability Smell of chemical on breath or clothes	**Refer for treatment as soon as possible** May need multiple diagnostic studies or procedures Monitor for changes in condition If vital signs abnormal, consider Level 2 Contact National Poison Control Center for advice (1-800-222-1222)
Level 4: Low Risk	Semi-Urgent
Moderate pain Poison oak or poison ivy exposure, urticaria, and rash	Reassess while waiting, per facility protocol Offer comfort measures May need simple diagnostic study or procedure Contact National Poison Control Center for advice (1-800-222-1222)
Level 5: Lower Risk	Nonurgent
Took twice the recommended amount of OTC medication Asymptomatic but parent or patient concerned	Reassess while waiting, per facility protocol Offer comfort measures May need examination only Contact National Poison Control Center for advice (1-800-222-1222) Online: www.webpoisoncontrol.org/

RELATED PROTOCOLS:
Alcohol and Drug Use, Abuse, Overdose, and Dependence • Bites, Insect and Tick • Bites, Marine Animal • Bites, Snake • Suicidal Behavior
See Appendices Q: Drugs of Abuse; R: Poisonings; S: Biological Agents/Chemical Agents

NOTES

_____
_____
_____
_____
_____

Pregnancy, Abdominal Pain

KEY QUESTIONS:

Name • Age • Onset • Allergies • Prior History • Severity • Pain Scale • Vital Signs • Oxygen
Saturation • Gestational Age • Recent Ultrasound • Number of Pregnancies

ACUITY LEVEL/ASSESSMENT	NURSING CONSIDERATIONS
Level 1: Critical	**Resuscitation**
Apnea or severe respiratory distress Imminent delivery, crowning noted Seizure Ruptured membranes with prolapsed cord Pale, diaphoretic, and lightheaded or weak	**Refer for immediate treatment** Staff at bedside Mobilization of resuscitation team Many resources needed Monitor fetal heart tones
Level 2: High Risk	**Emergent**
Altered mental status No fetal movement with gestational age >24 weeks Passing tissue with heavy vaginal bleeding Painful vaginal bleeding (abruptio placentae) and pregnancy >20 weeks Contractions every 2–3 minutes and pregnancy >20 weeks	**Do not delay treatment** Notify physician Multiple diagnostic studies or procedures Frequent consultation Continuous monitoring If pregnancy >20 weeks, transfer to labor and delivery, per facility protocol Monitor fetal heart tones
Level 3: Moderate Risk	**Urgent**
Painless vaginal bleeding (placenta previa) and pregnancy >20 weeks First trimester of pregnancy (ectopic) 20–37 weeks' gestation (preterm labor) Nausea, vomiting, diarrhea Bright red emesis, stools, or hematuria Sudden weight gain, edema, headache History of prior pregnancy complications Fever >102.2°F (>39.0°C)	**Refer for treatment as soon as possible** May need multiple diagnostic studies or procedures Monitor for changes in condition If vital signs abnormal, consider Level 2 Postural vital signs If pregnancy >20 weeks, transfer to labor and delivery, per facility protocol Monitor fetal heart tones

(continued)

Level 4: Low Risk	Semi-Urgent
Moderate pain Frequent urination or burning Fever, cough, earache, sore throat Vaginal discharge	Reassess while waiting, per facility protocol Offer comfort measures May need simple diagnostic study or procedure
Level 5: Lower Risk	Nonurgent
Heartburn "Morning sickness"	Reassess while waiting, per facility protocol Offer comfort measures May need examination only

RELATED PROTOCOLS:
Pregnancy, Back Pain • Pregnancy, Vaginal Bleeding • Pregnancy, Vaginal Discharge

NOTES

_____

_____

_____

_____

_____

_____

_____

_____

_____

_____

_____

_____

_____

_____

_____

_____

_____

_____

_____

_____

Pregnancy, Back Pain

KEY QUESTIONS:

Name • Age • Onset • Allergies • Prior History • Severity • Pain Scale • Vital Signs • Oxygen Saturation • Gestational Age • Recent Ultrasound • Number of Pregnancies

ACUITY LEVEL/ASSESSMENT	NURSING CONSIDERATIONS
Level 1: Critical	**Resuscitation**
Apnea or severe respiratory distress Unresponsive Imminent delivery, crowning noted Seizure Ruptured membranes with prolapsed cord Pale, diaphoretic, and lightheaded or weak	**Refer for immediate treatment** Staff at bedside Mobilization of resuscitation team Many resources needed Monitor fetal heart tones Place in knee-chest or Trendelenburg position Check cord for pulsation
Level 2: High Risk	**Emergent**
Altered mental status Contractions and <37 weeks' gestation No fetal movement Strong, regular contractions Recent trauma	**Do not delay treatment** Notify physician Multiple diagnostic studies or procedures Frequent consultation Continuous monitoring If pregnancy >20 weeks, transfer to labor and delivery, per facility protocol Monitor fetal heart tones
Level 3: Moderate Risk	**Urgent**
Fever >102.2°F (>39.0°C) Urinary frequency, burning, hematuria Difficulty starting a urine stream Flank pain Rectal pain Right upper quadrant pain or shoulder pain Multigravida and history of prior pregnancy complications	**Refer for treatment as soon as possible** May need multiple diagnostic studies or procedures Monitor for changes in condition If vital signs abnormal, consider Level 2 Orthostatic vital signs If pregnancy >20 weeks, transfer to labor and delivery, per facility protocol Monitor fetal heart tones

(continued)

Level 4: Low Risk	Semi-Urgent
Moderate pain Musculoskeletal pain	Reassess while waiting, per facility protocol Offer comfort measures May need simple diagnostic study or procedure
Level 5: Lower Risk	Nonurgent
Mild pain associated with increase in activity	Reassess while waiting, per facility protocol Offer comfort measures May need examination only

RELATED PROTOCOLS:
Pregnancy, Abdominal Pain • Pregnancy, Vaginal Bleeding • Pregnancy, Vaginal Discharge

NOTES

Pregnancy, Vaginal Bleeding

KEY QUESTIONS:
Name • Age • Onset • Allergies • Prior History • Severity • Pain Scale • Vital Signs • Last Menstrual Period/Gestational Age • Number of Regular-Size Saturated Pads • Medications

ACUITY LEVEL/ASSESSMENT	NURSING CONSIDERATIONS
Level 1: Critical	**Resuscitation**
Apnea or severe respiratory distress Pulseless Unresponsive Prolapsed cord Pale, diaphoretic, and lightheaded	**Refer for immediate treatment** Staff at bedside Mobilization of resuscitation team Many resources needed Monitor fetal heart tones Place in knee-chest or Trendelenburg position Check cord for pulsation
Level 2: High Risk	**Emergent**
Altered mental status Profuse, bright red blood and pregnancy >20 weeks Passing large clots or products of conception Painful vaginal bleeding (abruptio placentae) Hypotension or tachycardia Severe abdominal pain Lightheadedness No fetal movement and pregnancy >20 weeks Known trauma	**Do not delay treatment** Notify physician Multiple diagnostic studies or procedures Frequent consultation Continuous monitoring If pregnancy >20 weeks, transfer to labor and delivery, per facility protocol Monitor fetal heart tones Position patient on left side
Level 3: Moderate Risk	**Urgent**
Severe pain Painless vaginal bleeding and pregnancy >20 weeks Moderate flow, bright red blood (placenta previa)	**Refer for treatment as soon as possible** May need multiple diagnostic studies or procedures Monitor for changes in condition If vital signs abnormal, consider Level 2

(continued)

Level 3: Moderate Risk (*continued*)	Urgent
Strong, regular contractions Leaking clear fluid Less than 10 fetal movements in 1 hour	Postural vital signs If pregnancy >20 weeks, transfer to labor and delivery, per facility protocol Monitor fetal heart tones
Level 4: Low Risk	**Semi-Urgent**
Moderate pain Minimal bleeding but patient concerned	Reassess while waiting, per facility protocol Offer comfort measures May need simple diagnostic study or procedure
Level 5: Lower Risk	**Nonurgent**
Spotting dark brown or pink blood after intercourse	Reassess while waiting, per facility protocol Offer comfort measures May need examination only

RELATED PROTOCOLS:
Pregnancy, Abdominal Pain • Pregnancy, Back Pain • Pregnancy, Vaginal Discharge

NOTES

Pregnancy, Vaginal Discharge

KEY QUESTIONS:

Name • Age • Onset • Allergies • Prior History • Severity • Pain Scale • Vital Signs • Gestational Age • Medications

ACUITY LEVEL/ASSESSMENT	NURSING CONSIDERATIONS
Level 1: Critical	**Resuscitation**
Apnea or severe respiratory distress Pale, diaphoretic, and lightheaded or weak Ruptured membranes with prolapsed cord	**Refer for immediate treatment** Staff at bedside Mobilization of resuscitation team Many resources needed Monitor fetal heart tones Place in knee-chest or Trendelenburg position Check cord for pulsation
Level 2: High Risk	**Emergent**
Altered mental status Severe abdominal pain No fetal movement and pregnancy >20 weeks Imminent delivery with crowning or meconium	**Do not delay treatment** Notify physician Multiple diagnostic studies or procedures Frequent consultation Continuous monitoring If pregnancy >20 weeks, transfer to labor and delivery, per facility protocol Monitor fetal heart tones
Level 3: Moderate Risk	**Urgent**
Fever >102.2°F (>39.0°C) with purulent vaginal discharge Herpes outbreak with regular contractions or leaking of fluid Green, brown, or red-stained fluid	**Refer for treatment as soon as possible** May need multiple diagnostic studies or procedures Monitor for changes in condition If vital signs abnormal, consider Level 2 Monitor fetal heart tones

(continued)

Level 4: Low Risk	Semi-Urgent
Moderate pain Irregular contractions History of STD exposure Clumped, white, curd-like discharge Foul-smelling vaginal discharge	Reassess while waiting, per facility protocol Offer comfort measures May need simple diagnostic study or procedure
Level 5: Lower Risk	**Nonurgent**
Lost mucous plug Increase in vaginal mucus secretions	Reassess while waiting, per facility protocol Offer comfort measures May need examination only

RELATED PROTOCOLS:
Pregnancy, Vaginal Bleeding • Vaginal Bleeding, Abnormal

NOTES

_____

_____

_____

_____

_____

_____

_____

_____

_____

_____

_____

_____

_____

_____

_____

_____

_____

_____

Pregnancy, Vomiting

KEY QUESTIONS:
Name • Age • Onset • Allergies • Medications • Prior History • Severity • Pain Scale • Vital Signs • Gestational Age • Number of Pregnancies • Medications

ACUITY LEVEL/ASSESSMENT	NURSING CONSIDERATIONS
Level 1: Critical	**Resuscitation**
Severe respiratory distress Pale, diaphoretic, and lightheaded Unresponsive Pale, diaphoretic, dizzy, weak	**Refer for immediate treatment** Staff at bedside Mobilization of resuscitation team Many resources needed Monitor fetal heart tones
Level 2: High Risk	**Emergent**
Altered mental status Vomiting bright red blood Chest pain Difficulty breathing Recent head or abdominal trauma Abnormal vital signs	**Do not delay treatment** Notify physician Multiple diagnostic studies or procedures Frequent consultation Continuous monitoring Monitor fetal heart tones
Level 3: Moderate Risk	**Urgent**
Severe pain Signs of dehydration Coffee-grounds emesis Diabetes and hyperglycemia or hypoglycemia Lightheadedness Orthostatic vital signs Dark, amber-colored urine Right upper or lower quadrant pain	**Refer for treatment as soon as possible** May need multiple diagnostic studies or procedures Monitor for changes in condition Postural vital signs If vital signs abnormal, consider Level 2 Monitor fetal heart tones

(continued)

Level 3: Moderate Risk (*continued*)	Urgent
Abdominal pain and nausea, vomiting, or diarrhea Fever >102.2°F (>39.0°C) Tachycardia Hypotension	
Level 4: Low Risk	**Semi-Urgent**
Moderate pain Nausea and vomiting associated with gastroenteritis Vomiting >24 hours (no dehydration signs)	Reassess while waiting, per facility protocol Offer comfort measures May need simple diagnostic study or procedure
Level 5: Lower Risk	**Nonurgent**
Heartburn No other symptoms but patient concerned	Reassess while waiting, per facility protocol Offer comfort measures May need examination only

RELATED PROTOCOLS:
Pregnancy, Abdominal Pain • Vomiting

NOTES

_____

_____

_____

_____

_____

_____

_____

_____

_____

_____

_____

_____

Puncture Wound

KEY QUESTIONS:

Name • Age • Onset • Allergies • Medications • Prior History • Pain Scale • Vital Signs • Tetanus Immunization Status • Mechanism of Injury

ACUITY LEVEL/ASSESSMENT	NURSING CONSIDERATIONS
Level 1: Critical	**Resuscitation**
Apnea or severe respiratory distress Pulseless Unresponsive Involvement of vital organ Pale, diaphoretic, and lightheaded or weak	**Refer for immediate treatment** Staff at bedside Mobilization of resuscitation team Many resources needed
Level 2: High Risk	**Emergent**
Altered mental status High-risk mechanism of injury (mass, size, and velocity of wounding object and direction of impact) Large amount of bleeding and difficult to control with pressure Pulsatile bleeding Pulses absent distal to injury Skin cyanotic distal to wound High-pressure injection injury Impaled object obvious to head or trunk	**Do not delay treatment** Notify physician Multiple diagnostic studies or procedures Frequent consultation Continuous monitoring Leave impaled object in place Apply compression dressing to control bleeding Refer to appropriate mechanism of injury resource in Appendices M: Mechanisms of Injury: Adult; N: Mechanisms of Injury: School Age and Adolescent (7–17 years old); O: Mechanisms of Injury: Toddler and Preschooler (1–6 years old); P: Mechanisms of Injury: Infant (birth to 1 year old)
Level 3: Moderate Risk	**Urgent**
Severe pain Paresthesia distal to injury Pulses weak distal to injury Decreased range of motion to the affected area	**Refer for treatment as soon as possible** Reassess while waiting, per facility protocol May need multiple diagnostic studies or procedures

(continued)

Level 3: Moderate Risk (*continued*)	Urgent
Puncture wound in a joint Fever and chills History of bleeding disorder, cancer, etc. Tip of impaled object broken off and not visible Foreign body sensation persists Impaled object obvious to an extremity Wound contamination (dirty environment or object)	Monitor for changes in condition If vital signs abnormal, consider Level 2 Do not soak if wood sliver
Level 4: Low Risk	**Semi-Urgent**
Moderate pain Puncture wound through a shoe No prior tetanus prophylaxis Fever, red streaks, purulent drainage	Reassess while waiting, per facility protocol Offer comfort measures May need simple diagnostic study or procedure Do not soak if wood sliver
Level 5: Lower Risk	**Nonurgent**
Small object in distal extremity No other symptoms but parent or patient concerned Tetanus prophylaxis status > 5 years	Reassess while waiting, per facility protocol Offer comfort measures May need examination only Do not soak if wood sliver

RELATED PROTOCOLS:

Bites, Animal and Human • Bites, Marine Animal • Bites, Snake • Foreign Body, Skin • Laceration • Suicidal Behavior • Traumatic Injury • Wound Infection
See Appendices M: Mechanisms of Injury: Adult; N: Mechanisms of Injury: School Age and Adolescent (7–17 years old); O: Mechanisms of Injury: Toddler and Pre-schooler (1–6 years old); P: Mechanisms of Injury: Infant (birth to 1 year old)

NOTES

_____

_____

_____

_____

_____

_____

Rash, Adult and Pediatric

KEY QUESTIONS:

Name • Age • Onset • Allergies • Medications • Prior History • Pain Scale • Vital Signs • Oxygen Saturation • Number of Wet Diapers in an Infant • Recent Antibiotic History

ACUITY LEVEL/ASSESSMENT	NURSING CONSIDERATIONS
Level 1: Critical	**Resuscitation**
Severe respiratory distress Unresponsive Pale, diaphoretic, and lightheaded or weak Anaphylaxis Pulseless	**Refer for immediate treatment** Staff at bedside Mobilization of resuscitation team Many resources needed
Level 2: High Risk	**Emergent**
Altered mental status Fever and petechiae (nonblanching) or purpura (nonblanching) Fever and severe localized pain Red skin peeling off in sheets Stiff neck, severe headache Sudden onset of hives and difficulty breathing Child with any of the following: • Unusual drowsiness, refusal to drink, and noisy or fast breathing • Signs of dehydration: sunken eyes or fontanel, no wet diapers • Drooling • Rapidly progressing rash • At least two SIRS criteria: temperature >38.0°C or <36.0°C, HR >90, RR >20	**Do not delay treatment** Notify physician Multiple diagnostic studies or procedures Frequent consultation Continuous monitoring

(continued)

Level 3: Moderate Risk	Urgent
Severe pain Redness and swelling of the eyelid Facial swelling Fever, red rash, and using tampons or history of recent surgery Severe itching, irritation, and open skin	**Refer for treatment as soon as possible** Reassess while waiting, per facility protocol May need multiple diagnostic studies or procedures Monitor for changes in condition If vital signs abnormal, consider Level 2
Level 4: Low Risk	Semi-Urgent
Moderate pain Signs of infection: redness, swelling, pain, red streaks, or drainage from wound Fever, sore throat, or cold symptoms Joint pain or swelling Exposure to poison oak or poison ivy Localized area of painful blisters Nonlocalized fluid-filled blisters Newborn with blisters Blanching petechiae or purpura and no fever Multiple lesions in mouth Rash, blisters, pimples, or crusting under diaper area	Reassess while waiting, per facility protocol Offer comfort measures May need simple diagnostic study or procedure
Level 5: Lower Risk	Nonurgent
Dermatitis Herpes outbreak Asymptomatic rash lasting longer than 48 hours Recent exposure to chickenpox or measles Red or weeping rash in groin or diaper area Extensive rash, cause unknown	Reassess while waiting, per facility protocol Offer comfort measures May need examination only May isolate patients with communicable disease exposure and symptomatic from other waiting patients

RELATED PROTOCOLS:
Allergic Reaction • Bites, Animal and Human • Bites, Insect and Tick • Bites, Marine Animal • Bites, Snake • Poisoning, Exposure or Ingestion

NOTES

_____

_____

_____

_____

Rectal Problems

(see Foreign Body, Rectum or Vagina, for foreign body problem)

KEY QUESTIONS:

Name • Age • Onset • Allergies • Medications • Prior History • Severity • Pain Scale • Vital Signs

ACUITY LEVEL/ASSESSMENT	NURSING CONSIDERATIONS
Level 1: Critical	**Resuscitation**
Apnea or severe respiratory distress Pale, diaphoretic, and lightheaded or weak Unresponsive Pulseless	**Refer for immediate treatment** Staff at bedside Mobilization of resuscitation team Many resources needed
Level 2: High Risk	**Emergent**
Altered mental status Heavy rectal bleeding, mixed in the stool or passing of blood clots Traumatic injury to rectum by a knife or blunt object Black or bloody stools and lightheadedness Frequent black, tarry stools	**Do not delay treatment** Notify physician Multiple diagnostic studies or procedures Frequent consultation Continuous monitoring
Level 3: Moderate Risk	**Urgent**
Severe rectal pain Sexual assault Urinary retention Moderate rectal bleeding and no history of hemor-rhoids, or bleeding with constipation Acute abdominal pain, bloating, nausea, or vomiting Rectal pain and fever >102.2°F (>39.0°C) Foreign body in rectum Constipation and vomiting brown, yellow, or green bitter-tasting emesis Black or bloody stools and use of blood thinners, ste-roids, nonsteroidal anti-inflammatory medications, or large doses of aspirin Recent surgery (rectal, GI, GU, Gyn) Recent radiation treatments (rectal, prostate)	**Refer for treatment as soon as possible** May need multiple diagnostic studies or procedures Monitor for change in condition If vital signs abnormal, consider Level 2

(continued)

Level 4: Low Risk	Semi-Urgent
Moderate rectal pain or itching that interferes with activities of daily living Minimal rectal bleeding and history of hemorrhoids or bleeding with constipation Low-grade fever or signs of infection: spreading redness, open sores, drainage Exposure to an STD Painful blisters around rectal area Last bowel movement more than 5 days ago Infant with no stool for more than 6–10 days Fever, constipation, and history of recent surgery, injury, childbirth, or diverticulitis	Reassess while waiting, per facility protocol Offer comfort measures May need simple diagnostic study or procedure
Level 5: Lower Risk	Nonurgent
Worms visible in stool Rectal itching Chronic constipation Intermittent rectal pain with bowel movements	Reassess while waiting, per facility protocol Offer comfort measures May need examination only

RELATED PROTOCOLS:
Abdominal Pain, Adult • Abdominal Pain, Pediatric • Foreign Body, Rectum or Vagina • Sexual Assault

NOTES

_____

_____

_____

_____

_____

_____

_____

_____

_____

_____

Seizure

KEY QUESTIONS:

Name • Age • Onset • Allergies • Medications • Prior History • Severity • Pain Scale • Vital Signs • Oxygen Saturation • Drug or Alcohol Use • Traumatic Injury

ACUITY LEVEL/ASSESSMENT	NURSING CONSIDERATIONS
Level 1: Critical	**Resuscitation**
Apnea or severe respiratory distress Pulseless Unresponsive Status epilepticus Pale, diaphoretic, and lightheaded or weak	**Refer for immediate treatment** Staff at bedside Mobilization of resuscitation team Many resources needed
Level 2: High Risk	**Emergent**
Altered mental status History of head injury Pregnancy: eclampsia Overdose or poisoning Sudden onset of weakness, inability to move one side of the body, difficulty speaking, facial droop Strong suspicion of chemical exposure and symptomatic Severe headache First-time seizure Stroke signs/symptoms: sudden onset of facial droop, arm weakness, speech difficulty, severe headache, confusion, numbness, difficulty walking or seeing Persistent, unusual lethargy	**Do not delay treatment** Notify physician Multiple diagnostic studies or procedures Frequent consultation Continuous monitoring If multiple patients with similar symptoms or suspected chemical exposure, initiate decontamination procedures, per facility plan See Appendix S: Biological Agents/Chemical Agents

(continued)

Level 3: Moderate Risk	Urgent
Severe pain Fever >101.4°F (38.5°C) Sudden cessation of alcohol or drug consumption in the chronic user Frequent seizures while taking anticonvulsant medications Headache Nuchal rigidity History of seizures and inconsistent use of medications or excessive alcohol use	**Refer for treatment as soon as possible** May need multiple diagnostic studies or procedures Monitor for changes in condition If vital signs abnormal, consider Level 2
Level 4: Low Risk	Semi-Urgent
Moderate pain History of cancer, diabetes, or immunosuppression History of seizures and out of medication	Reassess while waiting, per facility protocol Offer comfort measures May need simple diagnostic study or procedure
Level 5: Lower Risk	Nonurgent
History of psychosomatic seizures History of seizures and alert and oriented after waking up from the seizure	Reassess while waiting, per facility protocol Offer comfort measures May need examination only

RELATED PROTOCOLS:
Alcohol and Drug Use, Abuse, Overdose, and Dependence • Altered Mental Status • Bites, Animal and Human • Bites, Insect and Tick • Bites, Marine Animal • Bites, Snake • Confusion • Diabetic Problems • Fever • Head Injury • Poisoning, Exposure or Ingestion • Traumatic Injury

NOTES

_____

_____

_____

_____

_____

_____

_____

_____

Seizure, Pediatric Febrile

KEY QUESTIONS:
Name • Age • Weight • Onset • Allergies • Prior History • Medications • Pain Scale • Vital Signs • Oxygen Saturation

ACUITY LEVEL/ASSESSMENT	NURSING CONSIDERATIONS
Level 1: Critical	**Resuscitation**
Apnea or severe respiratory distress Pulseless Unresponsive Status epilepticus Pale, diaphoretic, and lightheaded or weak	**Refer for immediate treatment** Staff at bedside Mobilization of resuscitation team Many resources needed
Level 2: High Risk	**Emergent**
Altered mental status Severe headache Stiff or painful neck Vomiting First-time seizure Child younger than 6 months or older than 5 years Fever >105°F (40.5°C)	**Do not delay treatment** Notify physician Multiple diagnostic studies or procedures Frequent consultation Continuous monitoring
Level 3: Moderate Risk	**Urgent**
Earache or respiratory infection unresponsive to antibiotics History of febrile seizures or high fever spikes Signs of dehydration: sunken eyes or fontanel, dry diaper Persistent fever >102°F (>38.9°C), unresponsive to fever-reducing measures	**Refer for treatment as soon as possible** May need multiple diagnostic studies or procedures Monitor for changes in condition If vital signs abnormal, consider Level 2 Apply cooling measures

(continued)

Level 4: Low Risk	Semi-Urgent
Feeding poorly Decreased fluid intake	Reassess while waiting, per facility protocol Offer comfort measures May need simple diagnostic study or procedure
Level 5: Lower Risk	Nonurgent
Alert and oriented after a seizure Afebrile with history of febrile seizures Child wants to sleep after seizure, but easily aroused without irritability	Reassess while waiting, per facility protocol Offer comfort measures May need examination only

RELATED PROTOCOLS:
Altered Mental Status • Confusion • Diabetic Problems • Fever • Head Injury •
Poisoning, Exposure or Ingestion • Traumatic Injury

NOTES

Sexual Assault

KEY QUESTIONS:

Name • Age • Onset • Allergies • Prior History • Pain Scale • Vital Signs • Oxygen Saturation • Mechanism of Injury • Last Menstrual Period • Last Consensual Intercourse • Gender Identification

ACUITY LEVEL/ASSESSMENT	NURSING CONSIDERATIONS
Level 1: Critical	**Resuscitation**
Apnea or severe respiratory distress Pulseless Unresponsive Pale, diaphoretic, and lightheaded or weak	**Refer for immediate treatment** Staff at bedside Mobilization of resuscitation team Many resources needed
Level 2: High Risk	**Emergent**
Altered mental status Profuse bleeding Genital trauma Multiple traumas from assault Head injury Difficulty breathing, chest pain, or abdominal pain Suspected fractures or dislocations Victim is a minor Suspicion of human trafficking	**Do not delay treatment** Notify physician Multiple diagnostic studies or procedures Frequent consultation Continuous monitoring
Level 3: Moderate Risk	**Urgent**
Severe pain Sexual assault <72 hours ago Severe anxiety Use of objects Possible exposure to date-rape drug Abrasions, lacerations, bruising, discoloration, or swelling Victim requests examination and collection of evidence	**Refer for treatment as soon as possible** May need multiple diagnostic studies or procedures Monitor for changes in condition If vital signs abnormal, consider Level 2 Sexual assault kit and sexual assault counselor, per facility protocol

(continued)

Level 4: Low Risk	Semi-Urgent
Moderate pain Sexual assault >72 hours ago	Reassess while waiting, per facility protocol Offer comfort measures May need simple diagnostic study or procedure Contact sexual assault counselor, per facility protocol
Level 5: Lower Risk	**Nonurgent**
Alleged assault without penetration	Reassess while waiting, per facility protocol Offer comfort measures May need examination only

RELATED PROTOCOLS:
Foreign Body, Rectum or Vagina • Rectal Problems • Traumatic Injury • Vaginal Bleeding, Abnormal

NOTES

_____

_____

_____

_____

_____

_____

_____

_____

_____

_____

_____

_____

_____

_____

_____

_____

_____

_____

Shoulder Pain

KEY QUESTIONS:

Name • Age • Onset • Allergies • Medications • Prior History • Pain Scale • Vital Signs • Oxygen Saturation • Traumatic Injury

ACUITY LEVEL/ASSESSMENT	NURSING CONSIDERATIONS
Level 1: Critical	**Resuscitation**
Apnea or severe respiratory distress Pulseless Unresponsive Pale, diaphoretic, and lightheaded or weak	**Refer for immediate treatment** Staff at bedside Mobilization of resuscitation team Many resources needed
Level 2: High Risk	**Emergent**
Altered mental status Pain radiates to chest, jaw, or neck Sudden onset, no known injury, and several cardiac risk factors present Difficulty breathing Decreased circulation in affected arm Open fracture	**Do not delay treatment** Notify physician Multiple diagnostic studies or procedures Frequent consultation Continuous monitoring
Level 3: Moderate Risk	**Urgent**
Severe pain Menstrual period more than 2–4 weeks late and abdominal pain present Fever and swollen, red, and tender joint Inability to raise arm above head Blunt trauma Decreased sensation in the affected arm	**Refer for treatment as soon as possible** May need multiple diagnostic studies or procedures Monitor for changes in condition Check capillary refill Monitor circulation, movement, and sensation of affected extremity If vital signs abnormal, consider Level 2

(continued)

Level 4: Low Risk	Semi-Urgent
Moderate pain Continued pain with decreased range of motion Recent injury and no reduction in pain after more than 3 days of ice, heat, and rest Discomfort in distal joints Recent abdominal surgery or diagnosis	Reassess while waiting, per facility protocol Offer comfort measures May need simple diagnostic study or procedure
Level 5: Lower Risk	Nonurgent
Chronic pain Discomfort increasing with activity Progressive joint pain and stiffness	Reassess while waiting, per facility protocol Offer comfort measures May need examination only

RELATED PROTOCOLS:
Chest Pain • Extremity Injury • Traumatic Injury

NOTES

_____

_____

_____

_____

_____

_____

_____

_____

_____

_____

_____

_____

_____

_____

Sinus Pain and Congestion

Name • Age • Onset • Allergies • Medications • Prior History • Severity • Pain Scale • Vital Signs • Oxygen Saturation

ACUITY LEVEL/ASSESSMENT	NURSING CONSIDERATIONS
Level 1: Critical	**Resuscitation**
Severe respiratory distress Pale, diaphoretic, and lightheaded or weak Unresponsive Pulseless	**Refer for immediate treatment** Staff at bedside Mobilization of resuscitation team Many resources needed
Level 2: High Risk	**Emergent**
Altered mental status Stiff neck and fever Wheezing with retractions Abnormal vital signs	**Do not delay treatment** Notify physician Multiple diagnostic studies or procedures Frequent consultation Continuous monitoring Provide IV access, per facility protocol Obtain laboratory samples, per facility protocol
Level 3: Moderate Risk	**Urgent**
Severe pain Severe headache or earache Fever >104°F (>40.0°C) and unresponsive to fever-reducing measures Mild wheezing Facial pain, swelling, redness, warmth, drainage, or fever Immunocompromised patient Fever >102°F (>39.0°C) and productive cough or shortness of breath	**Refer for treatment as soon as possible** May need multiple diagnostic studies or procedures Monitor for changes in condition If vital signs abnormal, consider Level 2

(continued)

Level 4: Low Risk	Semi-Urgent
Moderate pain Sore throat and persistent low-grade fever Headache worsening with movement Fever >101°F (>38.3°C) Green, brown, or yellow nasal discharge	Reassess while waiting, per facility protocol Offer comfort measures May need simple diagnostic study or procedure
Level 5: Lower Risk	Nonurgent
Sinus congestion Allergies Afebrile	Reassess while waiting, per facility protocol Offer comfort measures May need examination only

RELATED PROTOCOLS:
Cold Symptoms • Fever • Sore Throat

NOTES
_____
_____
_____
_____
_____
_____
_____
_____
_____
_____
_____
_____
_____
_____
_____
_____
_____
_____

Sore Throat

KEY QUESTIONS:

Name • Age • Onset • Allergies • Prior History • Associated Symptoms • Pain Scale • Vital Signs • Oxygen Saturation • Medications

ACUITY LEVEL/ASSESSMENT	NURSING CONSIDERATIONS
Level 1: Critical	**Resuscitation**
Severe respiratory distress Pale, diaphoretic, and lightheaded or weak Oxygen saturation <90% with oxygen	**Refer for immediate treatment** Many resources needed Staff at bedside Mobilization of resuscitation team
Level 2: High Risk	**Emergent**
Altered mental status Difficulty breathing (unrelated to nasal congestion) Excessive drooling in a child Stridor or inability to swallow own saliva Oxygen saturation <94% with oxygen Oxygen saturation <90% on room air "Kissing tonsils" and drooling	**Do not delay treatment** Notify physician Multiple diagnostic studies or procedures Frequent consultation Constant monitoring
Level 3: Moderate Risk	**Urgent**
Severe pain and difficulty swallowing Inability to open mouth completely Signs of dehydration Sore throat and lip or mouth swelling Neck pain or rigidity History of immunosuppression, age >60 years or diabetic, and fever >100.5°F (>38.1°C) History of rheumatic fever, mitral valve prolapse, or other heart problems "Kissing tonsils" and able to swallow own saliva	**Refer for treatment as soon as possible** May need multiple diagnostic studies or procedures Monitor for changes in condition If vital signs abnormal, consider Level 2 Rapid streptococcal test, per facility protocol

(continued)

Level 4: Low Risk	Semi-Urgent
Skin rash Exposure to streptococcal throat less than 2 weeks ago Moderate pain Hoarseness Yellow pus or white mucus at back of throat and fever Sore throat persists for more than 3 days Earache Red or enlarged tonsils	Reassess while waiting, per facility protocol Offer comfort measures May need a simple diagnostic study or procedure Rapid streptococcal test, per facility protocol
Level 5: Lower Risk	**Nonurgent**
Mild discomfort for less than 2 days Afebrile Chronic nasal congestion Coughing or sneezing with allergies	Reassess while waiting, per facility protocol Offer comfort measures May need examination only

RELATED PROTOCOLS:
Breathing Problems • Cold Symptoms • Cough • Ear Problems • Fever

NOTES

Stroke

KEY QUESTIONS:

Name • Age • Onset • Allergies • Medications • Prior History (Including Congestive Heart Failure, Stroke, Atrial Fibrillation, Coronary Artery Disease, Diabetes, Pulmonary Embolus, Deep Vein Thrombosis, etc.) • Pain Scale • Vital Signs • Duration of Symptoms • Implanted Devices (Pacemaker, Defibrillator, etc.)

ACUITY LEVEL/ASSESSMENT	NURSING CONSIDERATIONS
Level 1: Critical	**Resuscitation**
Severe respiratory distress Pale, diaphoretic, and lightheaded or weak Unresponsive	**Refer for immediate treatment** Staff at bedside Mobilization of resuscitation team Many resources needed
Level 2: High Risk	**Emergent**
Recreational street drug or prescription drug abuse in past 24 hours Rapid or irregular heart beat and dizziness or lightheadedness Facial droop Face, arm, or leg weakness or numbness Difficulty speaking or understanding others Confusion, severe headache, difficulty swallowing, or sudden change in vision Difficulty walking or maintaining balance Sudden memory loss or behavior change	**Do not delay treatment** Notify physician Multiple diagnostic studies or procedures Frequent consultation Continuous monitoring Continuous observation of suicidal patient
Level 3: Moderate Risk	**Urgent**
History of blood clots or heart problems Recent history of falls Temporary slurred speech or weakened grips Previous signs or symptoms that are now resolved	**Refer for treatment as soon as possible** May need multiple diagnostic studies or procedures Monitor for changes in condition If abnormal vital signs, consider Level 2

(continued)

Level 4: Low Risk	Semi-Urgent
Gradual onset of numbness, tingling, or burning sensation in extremities	Reassess while waiting, per facility protocol Offer comfort measures May need a simple diagnostic study or procedure
Level 5: Lower Risk	Nonurgent
Occasional weakness	Reassess while waiting, per facility protocol Offer comfort measures May need an examination only

RELATED PROTOCOLS:
Alcohol and Drug Use, Abuse, Overdose, and Dependence • Allergic Reaction • Altered Mental Status • Diabetic Problems • Headache • Head Injury • Heart Rate, Rapid • Heart Rate, Slow • Hypertension • Seizure • Weakness

NOTES

Suicidal Behavior

KEY QUESTIONS:
Name • Age • Onset • Allergies • Prior History • Pain Scale • Vital Signs • Oxygen Saturation • Prior Suicide Attempts and Methods

ACUITY LEVEL/ASSESSMENT	NURSING CONSIDERATIONS
Level 1: Critical	**Resuscitation**
Apnea or severe respiratory distress Pulseless Unresponsive Pale, diaphoretic, and lightheaded or weak	**Refer for immediate treatment** Staff at bedside Mobilization of resuscitation team Many resources needed
Level 2: High Risk	**Emergent**
Altered mental status Pulsatile bleeding from wounds Threat to self or others Overdose or poisoning Psychosis and potential harm to self or others Head trauma Hanging attempt and facial cyanosis, scleral hemorrhage, tongue swelling, petechiae, ligature marking Has a plan and the means to carry out the suicide	**Do not delay treatment** Notify physician Multiple diagnostic studies or procedures Frequent consultation Continuous monitoring Apply compression dressing to control bleeding Remove and check all clothing for weapons or means to commit suicide
Level 3: Moderate Risk	**Urgent**
Severe pain Refusal to talk, withdrawn, or no eye contact History of prior attempts Depression Intoxication	**Refer for treatment as soon as possible** May need multiple diagnostic studies or procedures Maintain constant supervision of patient Monitor for changes in condition If vital signs abnormal, consider Level 2 Contact crisis personnel or social worker, per facility protocol

(continued)

Level 4: Low Risk	Semi-Urgent
Moderate pain Suicidal thoughts with no plans Stopped taking medication	Reassess while waiting, per facility protocol Offer comfort measures May need simple diagnostic study or procedure Observe while waiting Contact crisis personnel or social worker, per facility protocol
Level 5: Lower Risk	Nonurgent
History of depression controlled with medication	Reassess while waiting, per facility protocol Offer comfort measures May need examination only

RELATED PROTOCOLS:
Anxiety • Depression • Poisoning, Exposure or Ingestion

NOTES

Sunburn

Name • Age • Onset • Allergies • Medications • Prior History • Severity • Pain Scale • Vital Signs • Tetanus Immunization Status

ACUITY LEVEL/ASSESSMENT	NURSING CONSIDERATIONS
Level 1: Critical	**Resuscitation**
Severe respiratory distress Unresponsive Pale, diaphoretic, and lightheaded or weak Hypotension, tachycardia	**Refer for immediate treatment** Many resources needed Staff at bedside Mobilization of resuscitation team
Level 2: High Risk	**Emergent**
Altered mental status Temperature >104.9°F (>40.5°C) and unresponsive to cooling measures Dry, hot skin and lightheadedness Diaphoresis, cool skin, and lightheadedness Facial swelling	**Do not delay treatment** Notify physician Multiple diagnostic studies or procedures Frequent consultation Continuous monitoring Perform cooling measures Provide IV access, per facility protocol
Level 3: Moderate Risk	**Urgent**
Severe pain Visual changes and/or severe eye pain Signs of dehydration Vomiting Circumferential burns around extremities, digits, or genitals Large area of blistered skin	**Refer for treatment as soon as possible** May need multiple diagnostic studies or procedures Monitor for changes in condition If vital signs abnormal, consider Level 2

(continued)

Level 4: Low Risk	Semi-Urgent
Moderate pain Small areas of blisters Open blisters Red streaks extending from blistered area Tetanus immunization more than 5 years ago	Reassess while waiting, per facility protocol Offer comfort measures May need simple diagnostic study or procedure
Level 5: Lower Risk	Nonurgent
Mild sunburn Sunburn responsive to over-the-counter analgesics	Reassess while waiting, per facility protocol May need examination only Offer comfort measures

RELATED PROTOCOLS:
Burns • Heat Exposure • Lightheadedness/Fainting

NOTES

_____

_____

_____

_____

_____

_____

_____

_____

_____

_____

_____

_____

_____

_____

_____

_____

_____

Toothache/Tooth Injury

KEY QUESTIONS:

Name • Age • Onset • Allergies • Medications • Prior History • Severity • Pain Scale • Vital Signs • Piercings • Injury or Assault

ACUITY LEVEL/ASSESSMENT	NURSING CONSIDERATIONS
Level 1: Critical	**Resuscitation**
Severe respiratory distress Pale, diaphoretic, and lightheaded or weak Unresponsive Pulseless	**Refer for immediate treatment** Many resources needed Staff at bedside Mobilization of resuscitation team
Level 2: High Risk	**Emergent**
Altered mental status Traumatic dental injuries with risk of airway compromise or neck injury Gnawing pain in lower teeth and chest, neck, shoulder, or arm Similar pain in the past and related to a heart problem Tooth knocked out Bleeding uncontrolled with constant pressure	**Do not delay treatment** Notify physician Multiple diagnostic studies or procedures Frequent consultation Continuous monitoring Tooth needs to be placed in socket ASAP; minutes count
Level 3: Moderate Risk	**Urgent**
Severe pain Facial pain, swelling, redness, warmth, drainage, or fever Fever >104°F (>40.0°C) and unresponsive to fever-reducing measures History of cardiac valve replacement Fever and neck pain Severe swelling of oral tissue Use of bisphosphonates	**Refer for treatment as soon as possible** May need multiple diagnostic studies or procedures Monitor for changes in condition If vital signs abnormal, consider Level 2

(continued)

Level 4: Low Risk	Semi-Urgent
Moderate pain Swollen painful gums Purulent drainage Foul taste or odor in mouth Recent dental work in painful area Chipped or fractured tooth	Reassess while waiting, per facility protocol Offer comfort measures May need simple diagnostic study or procedure
Level 5: Lower Risk	Nonurgent
Sores in mouth Loose or decayed tooth Sensitive to heat, cold, or pressure Tooth discolored	Reassess while waiting, per facility protocol May need examination only Offer comfort measures

RELATED PROTOCOLS:
Mouth Problems • Traumatic Injury

NOTES

_____

_____

_____

_____

_____

_____

_____

_____

_____

_____

_____

_____

_____

_____

_____

_____

_____

_____

Traumatic Injury
(Skateboard, Ski, Snowboard, Bike, Car, etc.)

KEY QUESTIONS:

Name • Age • Onset • Allergies • Prior History • Severity • Pain Scale • Vital Signs • Oxygen Saturation • Extent of Injuries • Mechanism of Injury • Use of Safety Equipment

ACUITY LEVEL/ASSESSMENT	NURSING CONSIDERATIONS
Level 1: Critical	**Resuscitation**
Apnea or severe respiratory distress Pulseless Unresponsive High-risk mechanism of injury Pale, diaphoretic, and lightheaded or weak	**Refer for immediate treatment** Staff at bedside Mobilization of resuscitation team C-spine immobilization Many resources needed
Level 2: High Risk	**Emergent**
Altered mental status Uncontrolled bleeding High rate of speed Unrestrained in vehicle Bruising over vital organs Multiple large lacerations Point tenderness High-risk medical history (diabetes, cancer, hemophilia, etc.)	**Do not delay treatment** Notify physician Multiple diagnostic studies or procedures Frequent consultation Continuous monitoring C-spine immobilization
Level 3: Moderate Risk	**Urgent**
Severe pain Ambulatory at scene of the traumatic injury Small lacerations with bleeding controlled Moderate-risk mechanism of injury	**Refer for treatment as soon as possible** May need multiple diagnostic studies or procedures Monitor for changes in condition If vital signs abnormal, consider Level 2

(continued)

Level 4: Low Risk	Semi-Urgent
Moderate pain Minor bruising or aches Minor lacerations or abrasions with bleeding controlled If other occupant of same vehicle was a fatality, consider Level 3	Reassess while waiting, per facility protocol Offer comfort measures May need simple diagnostic study or procedure
Level 5: Lower Risk	Nonurgent
No complaints of pain, bruising, or injury from a low-speed, minor MVA or traumatic injury More than 24 hours since traumatic injury	Reassess while waiting, per facility protocol Offer comfort measures May need examination only

RELATED PROTOCOLS:
Ankle Pain and Swelling • Back Pain • Cold Exposure, Hypothermia/Frostbite • Extremity Injury • Head Injury • Knee Pain and/or Swelling • Neck Pain • Puncture Wound • Shoulder Pain

See Appendices L: MVA Triage Questions; M: Mechanisms of Injury: Adult; N: Mechanisms of Injury: School Age and Adolescent (7–17 years old); O: Mechanisms of Injury: Toddler and Preschooler (1–6 years old); P: Mechanisms of Injury: Infant (birth to 1 year old)

NOTES

Urinary Catheter Problems

KEY QUESTIONS:

Name • Age • Onset • Allergies • Medications • Prior History • Severity • Pain Scale • Vital Signs • Date Catheter Inserted

ACUITY LEVEL/ASSESSMENT	NURSING CONSIDERATIONS
Level 1: Critical	**Resuscitation**
Severe respiratory distress Pale, diaphoretic, and lightheaded or weak Pulseless Unresponsive	**Refer for immediate treatment** Staff at bedside Mobilization of resuscitation team Many resources needed
Level 2: High Risk	**Emergent**
Altered mental status Severe flank, abdominal, or back pain and fever >102°F (>39.0°C) Profuse bright red blood from catheter	**Do not delay treatment** Notify physician Multiple diagnostic studies or procedures Frequent consultation Continuous monitoring
Level 3: Moderate Risk	**Urgent**
Severe pain Gross hematuria Passing clots through catheter Painful, distended bladder No urine output for more than 8 hours At least two SIRS criteria: temperature >38.0°C or <36.0°C, HR >90, RR >20 Surgically placed catheter or tube displaced	**Refer for treatment as soon as possible** May need multiple diagnostic studies or procedures Monitor for changes in condition If vital signs abnormal, consider Level 2

(continued)

Level 4: Low Risk	Semi-Urgent
Moderate pain Recent urologic surgery Taking a blood-thinning agent and urine pink or red Skin irritation near meatus Cloudy, foul-smelling urine Fever >100.4°F (>38.0°C)	Reassess while waiting, per facility protocol Offer comfort measures May need simple diagnostic study or procedure
Level 5: Lower Risk	Nonurgent
Catheter leak Mild discomfort	Reassess while waiting, per facility protocol Offer comfort measures May need examination only

RELATED PROTOCOLS:
Abdominal Pain, Adult • Abdominal Pain, Pediatric • Fever • Urination Problems

NOTES

_____

_____

_____

_____

_____

_____

_____

_____

_____

_____

_____

_____

_____

_____

_____

_____

_____

Urination Problems

Name • Age • Onset • Allergies • Medications • Prior History • Severity • Pain Scale • Vital Signs

ACUITY LEVEL/ASSESSMENT	NURSING CONSIDERATIONS
Level 1: Critical	**Resuscitation**
Severe respiratory distress Pale, diaphoretic, and lightheaded or weak Pulseless Unresponsive	**Refer for immediate treatment** Staff at bedside Mobilization of resuscitation team Many resources needed
Level 2: High Risk	**Emergent**
Altered mental status Severe abdominal pain with fever >102°F (>39.0°C) Hematuria and flank trauma, history of renal transplant, or severe abdominal or flank pain Severe abdominal pain and unable to void for more than 8 hours or catheter bag empty for more than 8 hours Traumatic injury to urethra and unable to stop bleeding with pressure	**Do not delay treatment** Notify physician Multiple diagnostic studies or procedures Frequent consultation Continuous monitoring
Level 3: Moderate Risk	**Urgent**
Severe pain Fever >102°F (>39.0°C) Persistent flank, back, or abdominal pain Hematuria and colicky flank pain or use of anticoagulants Pain with urination, back or flank pain, and fever >100.5°F (>38.1°C)	**Refer for treatment as soon as possible** May need multiple diagnostic studies or procedures Monitor for changes in condition If vital signs abnormal, consider Level 2 Urine sample and dipstick, per facility protocol

(continued)

Level 3: Moderate Risk (*continued*)	Urgent
Pain or bleeding and history of diabetes or immunosuppression New onset of incontinence History of renal or prostate disease Recent trauma (back, abdominal, genital area) Unable to urinate for more than 4–8 hours Recent urinary or abdominal surgery and dysuria Use of erectile dysfunction medications Priapism for more than 3 hours Pregnant and unable to void Rectal pain	
Level 4: Low Risk	**Semi-Urgent**
Moderate pain Fever >100.4°F (>38.0°C) Nausea or vomiting Genital herpes or STD Difficulty urinating after sexual intercourse Urinary frequency, urgency, and/or hematuria Full bladder and unable to urinate for less than 4 hours	Reassess while waiting, per facility protocol Offer comfort measures May need simple diagnostic study or procedure Urine sample and dipstick, per facility protocol
Level 5: Lower Risk	**Nonurgent**
Burning sensation after exposure to bubble baths, nylon underwear, soaps, or other products applied to the perineal area Urinary frequency or fullness Nocturia	Reassess while waiting, per facility protocol Offer comfort measures May need examination only

RELATED PROTOCOLS:
Abdominal Pain, Adult • Abdominal Pain, Pediatric • Back Pain • Fever • Urinary Catheter Problems

NOTES

_____

_____

_____

_____

_____

Vaginal Bleeding, Abnormal

KEY QUESTIONS:
Name • Age • Onset • Allergies • Medications • Prior History • Severity • Pain Scale •
Vital Signs • Birth Control Measures • Last Menstrual Period • Number of Pregnancies

ACUITY LEVEL/ASSESSMENT	NURSING CONSIDERATIONS
Level 1: Critical	**Resuscitation**
Severe respiratory distress Pale, diaphoretic, and lightheaded or weak Pulseless Unresponsive	**Refer for immediate treatment** Staff at bedside Mobilization of resuscitation team Many resources needed
Level 2: High Risk	**Emergent**
Altered mental status Sexual assault and profuse bleeding or injury with an object Profuse bleeding saturating more than three full-size pads/hour Passing products of conception Diaphoretic History of blood disorders Pregnancy >20 weeks' gestation Hypotension Vaginal bleeding, abdominal or shoulder pain, last period 2–4 weeks late, and possibility of pregnancy Retained foreign object	**Do not delay treatment** Notify physician Multiple diagnostic studies or procedures Frequent consultation Continuous monitoring
Level 3: Moderate Risk	**Urgent**
Severe pain Nausea, vomiting, or lightheadedness Increased thirst or signs of dehydration	**Refer for treatment as soon as possible** May need multiple diagnostic studies or procedures

(*continued*)

Level 3: Moderate Risk (*continued*)	Urgent
Increased abdominal pain with movement Orthostatic changes Recent abortion or miscarriage with fever, pain, and increasing bleeding Abdominal trauma, assault, MVA, fall, etc. Suspicion of human trafficking	Monitor for changes in condition If vital signs abnormal, consider Level 2 Measure orthostatic vital signs
Level 4: Low Risk	**Semi-Urgent**
Moderate pain Cramping Heavier-than-normal period Bleeding increased with increase in activity or change in birth control pills Bleeding for more than 10 days	Reassess while waiting, per facility protocol Offer comfort measures May need simple diagnostic study or procedure
Level 5: Lower Risk	**Nonurgent**
Spotty bleeding after sexual intercourse Recently started taking oral contraceptives Normal menses Patient concerned about menopause or pregnancy	Reassess while waiting, per facility protocol Offer comfort measures May need examination only

RELATED PROTOCOLS:
Foreign Body, Rectum or Vagina ● Pregnancy, Vaginal Discharge

NOTES

_____

_____

_____

_____

_____

_____

_____

_____

_____

_____

Vomiting

KEY QUESTIONS:
Name • Age • Onset • Allergies • Medications • Prior History • Severity • Pain Scale • Vital Signs • Health of Other Household Members • Recent Trauma

ACUITY LEVEL/ASSESSMENT	NURSING CONSIDERATIONS
Level 1: Critical	**Resuscitation**
Severe respiratory distress Pale, diaphoretic, and lightheaded or weak Unresponsive Pulseless	**Refer for immediate treatment** Staff at bedside Mobilization of resuscitation team Many resources needed
Level 2: High Risk	**Emergent**
Altered mental status Head injury Persistent vomiting of frank blood or coffee-grounds emesis Chest, jaw, or arm pain Abdominal trauma Diabetic and glucose >400 mg/dL	**Do not delay treatment** Notify physician Multiple diagnostic studies or procedures Frequent consultation Continuous monitoring
Level 3: Moderate Risk	**Urgent**
Severe abdominal pain or headache for more than 2 hours Signs of dehydration Possible ingestion of or exposure to poisonous substance History of diabetes, cancer, other chronic illness, or immunosuppression Age >60 years and vomited more than once Fever >104°F (>40°C) Changes in orthostatic vital signs	**Refer for treatment as soon as possible** May need multiple diagnostic studies or procedures Monitor for changes in condition If abnormal vital signs, consider Level 2

(continued)

Level 4: Low Risk	Semi-Urgent
Moderate pain Recent ingestion of an antibiotic, pain medication, or new medication Vomiting for more than 48 hours	Reassess while waiting, per facility protocol Offer comfort measures May need a simple diagnostic study or procedure
Level 5: Lower Risk	Nonurgent
Vomiting for less than 24 hours Recent surgery, hospitalization, or diagnostic procedure Other household members are ill Excessive ingestion of food, alcohol, or fluids Possible pregnancy	Reassess while waiting, per facility protocol Offer comfort measures May need an examination only

RELATED PROTOCOLS:
Abdominal Pain, Adult • Abdominal Pain, Pediatric • Diarrhea, Adult • Diarrhea, Pediatric • Fever • Head Injury • Poisoning, Exposure or Ingestion • Pregnancy, Vomiting • Traumatic Injury

NOTES
_____
_____
_____
_____
_____
_____
_____
_____
_____
_____
_____
_____
_____
_____
_____

Weakness

KEY QUESTIONS:

Name • Age • Onset • Allergies • Medications • Prior History • Severity • Vital Signs • Oxygen Saturation • Pain Scale

ACUITY LEVEL/ASSESSMENT	NURSING CONSIDERATIONS
Level 1: Critical	**Resuscitation**
Apnea or severe respiratory distress Unresponsive Pale, diaphoretic, and lightheaded or weak Pulseless	**Refer for immediate treatment** Staff at bedside Mobilization of resuscitation team Many resources needed
Level 2: High Risk	**Emergent**
Sudden onset or persistent altered mental status Drug or alcohol overdose Inability to stand, walk, or bear weight Severe headache Chest pain Rapid heartbeat with syncope/diaphoresis Sudden onset of weakness to one side of the body Weakness in face, arm, or leg Visual disturbances Temporary slurred speech or weakened grip Speech and language problems Irregular pulse Severe abdominal pain Loss of movement in arms or legs, confusion, difficulty speaking, numbness or tingling, or blurred vision, and onset less than 2 hours Hand or foot cold or blue Headache, fever, and stiff or painful neck Changes in orthostatic vital signs	**Do not delay treatment** Notify physician Multiple diagnostic studies or procedures Frequent consultation Continuous monitoring Fingerstick glucose

(continued)

Level 3: Moderate Risk	Urgent
Recent head injury or trauma (rule out head bleed) Persistent high fever Severe abdominal pain and normal vital signs Temporary slurred speech or weakened grips Pain, swelling, warmth, or redness in affected limb Severe pain interfering with normal activity Immunocompromised	**Refer for treatment as soon as possible** May need multiple diagnostic studies or procedures Monitor for changes in condition If vital signs abnormal, consider Level 2
Level 4: Low Risk	**Semi-Urgent**
History of dieting or use of diuretics Gradual onset of numbness, tingling, or burning sensation in extremities Pain radiates to arm or leg Fever; cough; green, yellow, or brown sputum; body aches for more than 24 hours; and unresponsive to home care measures History of taking cholesterol-lowering medication Recent history of frequent falls	Reassess while waiting, per facility protocol Offer comfort measures May need a simple diagnostic study or procedure
Level 5: Lower Risk	**Nonurgent**
Exhaustion Occasional weakness History of neuromuscular problems that are unresponsive to medication Increased exercise, activity level, or stress History of muscular pain	Reassess while waiting, per facility protocol Offer comfort measures May need examination only

RELATED PROTOCOLS:
Altered Mental Status • Breathing Problems • Chest Pain • Fever • Headache • Stroke

For chest pain, see Chest Pain; for difficulty breathing, see Breathing Problems; for altered mental status, see Altered Mental Status

NOTES

_____

_____

_____

_____

_____

Wound Infection

KEY QUESTIONS:
Name • Age • Onset • Allergies • Medications • Prior History • Severity • Pain Scale • Vital Signs

ACUITY LEVEL/ASSESSMENT	NURSING CONSIDERATIONS
Level 1: Critical	Resuscitation
Severe respiratory distress Pale, diaphoretic, and lightheaded or weak Unresponsive Pulseless	**Refer for immediate treatment** Staff at bedside Mobilization of resuscitation team Many resources needed
Level 2: High Risk	Emergent
Altered mental status Sutured or stapled wound >50% open	**Do not delay treatment** Notify physician Multiple diagnostic studies or procedures Frequent consultation Continuous monitoring
Level 3: Moderate Risk	Urgent
Severe pain Surgical wound dehiscence Purulent drainage Fever Swollen lymph nodes Red streaking away from the wound Headache or general illness High-risk history (e.g., diabetes, immunosuppression, chronic illness, chemotherapy, use of steroids) and wound not healing well	**Refer for treatment as soon as possible** May need multiple diagnostic studies or procedures Monitor for changes in condition If abnormal vital signs, consider Level 2

(continued)

Level 4: Low Risk	Semi-Urgent
Moderate pain	Reassess while waiting, per facility protocol Offer comfort measures May need a simple diagnostic study or procedure
Level 5: Lower Risk	Nonurgent
Wound itching Tetanus immunization more than 5 years ago	Reassess while waiting, per facility protocol Offer comfort measures May need an examination only

RELATED PROTOCOLS:
Abdominal Pain, Adult • Abdominal Pain, Pediatric • Diabetic Problems

NOTES

Wrist Pain and Swelling

KEY QUESTIONS:

Name • Age • Onset • Allergies • Medications • Prior History • Severity • Pain Scale •
Vital Signs • Mechanism of Injury

ACUITY LEVEL/ASSESSMENT	NURSING CONSIDERATIONS
Level 1: Critical	**Resuscitation**
Severe respiratory distress Pale, diaphoretic, and lightheaded or weak Unresponsive	**Refer for immediate treatment** Staff at bedside Mobilization of resuscitation team Many resources needed
Level 2: High Risk	**Emergent**
Altered mental status Pulsatile bleeding No radial pulse Cyanosis of the hand Open fracture Suicidal behavior High-pressure injection injury	**Do not delay treatment** Notify physician Multiple diagnostic studies or procedures Frequent consultation Continuous monitoring Continuous observation of suicidal patient
Level 3: Moderate Risk	**Urgent**
Severe pain Unsplinted angulated deformity Wrist swollen to twice its normal size Fever, drainage, red streaks Impaled object Bite wound	**Refer for treatment as soon as possible** May need multiple diagnostic studies or procedures Monitor for changes in condition If abnormal vital signs, consider Level 2

(continued)

Level 4: Low Risk	Semi-Urgent
Moderate pain Splinted deformity High-risk mechanism of injury Decreased mobility Inability to make a fist Retained foreign body Point tenderness	Reassess while waiting, per facility protocol Offer comfort measures May need a simple diagnostic study or procedure
Level 5: Lower Risk	Nonurgent
Pain, swelling, or discoloration Chronic discomfort (old injury) History of arthritis or tendonitis Pain increasing with repetitive activities	Reassess while waiting, per facility protocol Offer comfort measures May need an examination only

RELATED PROTOCOLS:
Extremity Injury • Shoulder Pain • Traumatic Injury

NOTES

_____

_____

_____

_____

_____

_____

_____

_____

_____

_____

_____

_____

_____

_____

_____

_____

APPENDIX A

Triage Program Development

Introduction

This appendix provides a comprehensive guide for the development of a formal triage program that can be used in larger urban EDs, smaller community hospitals, urgent care centers, and rural or remote healthcare centers. It can also be used in the development of a triage unit established in response to a multiple casualty event (MCE) caused by fires, utility failures, severe weather, pandemics, terrorist incidents, chemical spills, active shooter incidents, or any other event with a large influx of victims needing rapid triage to assess the severity of symptoms and need for timely care. In developing an effective triage program, the following issues should be addressed:

- The triage area/station
- Patient flow
- Safety
- Supplies and equipment
- Rural and remote triage
- Legal considerations
- Maintaining quality
- Training
- Managing mass casualties and active shooter incidents

The Triage Area/Station

Establish a triage station that is clearly identified. On entering a facility, patients will generally seek out the first person they see unless there is clear signage to give specific direction where to go: **Emergency patients see triage nurse** with an arrow pointing to the triage station or **Wait here for next triage nurse.**

- It is natural to go directly to a window or counter with a person who looks available to help. Some EDs place a registration person at the first contact point to enter patients into the computer system and then direct them to the triage nurse before any financial information is obtained.
- The triage area should include a counter or window for the rapid triage or first encounter.
- Establish a more private area for a more comprehensive triage assessment.

- EDs seeing more than 30,000 patients a year will need at least two persons stationed at triage: either two triage nurses or one triage nurse and a technician.
- The initial rapid triage station should provide seating for the nurse and for patients unable to stand at a counter.
- The comprehensive triage area should provide seating for both the nurse and the patient. Some nurses prefer to use a stand-up computer terminal while assessing the patient.
- If more than five patients are waiting for a comprehensive triage for more than 15 minutes, consider adding a second nurse and workspace to conduct the triage assessment. A patient's condition could have deteriorated if waiting for an hour for a comprehensive assessment.
- Establish a seating area adjacent to the initial rapid triage station to place urgent patients and others the nurse is concerned about so that the patient is always visible to the triage nurse. Some facilities require a reassessment for any urgent patient waiting for more than 60 minutes.
- Develop a system for keeping track of where patients are in the triage process and the next step from triage to treatment. Some EDs use chart racks and move the chart from one rack to another as each phase of the process is completed, such as waiting for a comprehensive triage, registration, nurse-initiated/technician orders for treatment, laboratory or x-ray orders (per facility policy and procedures), and ready for next available treatment bed. This system can also be maintained on an electronic tracking system so that staff in the treatment area are also familiar with the flow of patients through triage.
- Establish more than one exit route out of each triage station.

Patient Flow

- Most EDs use a staged approach to triage including a rapid triage nurse, a comprehensive assessment nurse, a technician, and patient registration.
- Rapid triage starts across the room when the person enters the facility. The RN obtains the patient's name, date of birth (DOB), chief complaint, and time of arrival, and then makes a decision to move the patient to a treatment area for emergent care or the second stage, which may be registration or a comprehensive triage for a more thorough assessment. The rapid triage can occur at an open counter easily accessed by the patient. Rapid triage takes about 60 to 90 seconds and is a quick method to identify people at greatest risk of deterioration while waiting for the more in-depth triage.
  - Assess for potential life-threatening conditions.
  - Assess mobility: Does the person use an assistive device such as crutches, walker, cane, or wheelchair? Is his or her gait fast, slow, or weakened, or is the person unable to ambulate?

- Assess facial expression or body language, which can indicate discomfort, fear, pain, facial drooping, signs of a stroke, or aggressive behavior.
- Assess mental status: Is the person altered or impaired?
- Assess airway/breathing: Is it labored, noisy? Does the person seem to have difficulty breathing, getting air in or out? Is the person drooling?
- Assess circulation, note the color of the skin (pale, blue, red), is the person diaphoretic, is there obvious bleeding?
- Assess neurologic status, note the level of responsiveness and upper and lower extremity movement and strength.
- Assess signs of environmental exposure due to weather, chemicals, fire.

- The comprehensive triage should occur in a more private area and includes vital signs including oxygen saturation, and a more comprehensive assessment to determine acuity and urgency for treatment.
- If the RN is busy completing a comprehensive assessment, a technician can meet and greet the patient, determine the chief complaint, name, and DOB, and reassure the patient that the nurse will be available shortly. If the complaint seems urgent and the triage RN cannot be interrupted, an RN from the treatment area should complete the triage to determine if emergent care is appropriate.
- Technicians can play a valuable role at triage. Responsibilities may include the following:
  - Measure vital signs
  - Help facilitate patient movement through the triage process
  - Collect some patient history
  - Perform laboratory testing per facility policy such as blood draws
  - Conduct EKGs per facility policy
  - Apply dressings or splints
  - Assist patients with mobility (i.e., assist in and out of cars, provide wheel chairs)
  - Keep the triage area stocked with supplies and equipment
  - Be familiar with conditions that often require immediate attention
- Some EDs also utilize advance care providers at triage to help decrease waits and utilize the ED more efficiently. This role may be filled by an MD, NP, or PA who can provide a medical screening exam (MSE) at triage to determine that the person does not have an emergency medical condition and can be safely referred to other healthcare resources. (See Legal Considerations later in this appendix for additional information on the MSE.)

Safety at Triage

- Staff must know the exit route plan to avoid entrapment by hostile or violent patients or visitors.
- Install a panic button to alert security or the police that there is a threat at triage. Train staff and ensure that all staff members know the location and purpose of the panic button.
- If the ED doors are not always locked on closing, install a lock-down button at triage to prevent hostile persons from entering the ED treatment areas.
- Install cameras with screens in the ED/security so that the triage area is visible to other staff/security at all times.
- Train staff in communication techniques and managing aggressive behaviors.
- Place security at triage or maintain a security presence by security frequently circulating through the triage area.
- See "Prepare for and Manage Active Shooter Incidents" section in this appendix for additional information and safety measures to take before and during a violent event.

Triage Supplies and Equipment

- Emergency equipment: oral airways, bag-valve mask, crash cart
- Mechanism to obtain immediate assistance in the event of a code blue or a potentially violent or threatening situation. May include a panic button, radio, cell or regular phone, computer tracking system, or intercom.
- Stabilization or immobilization equipment; backboards, splints, C-collars
- EKG machine
- EKG monitor
- Vital sign devices: thermometers (electronic for rapid read-out), blood pressure cuffs of all sizes (pediatric, small, medium, large, and extra large), pulse oximeter
- Blood glucose measurement device
- Emesis basins/bags, specimen cups with labels, gauze—multiple sizes, saline, instant ice packs or ice bags if ice machine readily available, slings
- Personal protective equipment: gloves (multiple sizes), gowns, masks, hand sanitizers
- Backup paper forms are critical if the computer system is unavailable. Paper forms may include laboratory slips, order forms, paper charts for documentation of assessment and treatment, consent forms.

Rural and Remote Triage

Healthcare facilities and a variety of healthcare services may have diminished resources because of their remoteness but still have to provide triage to establish the severity of illness and need for timely treatment. This second edition of *Emergency Nursing 5-Tier Triage* provides the tools, triage protocols, and guidelines to assist in providing safe and comprehensive triage service in any setting. Elements to consider include the following:

- Facility or service may not have medical staff onsite.
- Nurses must rely on their assessment skills, judgment, and experience.
- Facility may not have the support and response of a multidisciplinary team. Staff members may have multiple roles; respiratory therapy, laboratories, radiology imaging, IV therapy, etc.
- Facility often relies on local practice and treatment guidelines.
- Emphasis is on time to treatment rather than time to be seen by a provider.
- Triage often involves more than assessment of acuity, can involve early medical management decisions and treatment.
- Rural nurse may have multiple jobs within a facility and may not consistently serve in the triage nurse position.
- Facility may lack the safety factor of having others around to provide support and advice.
- There may be a lack of other viable options for care. If transfer to a higher level of care is necessary, must consider the distance and safest way to travel. Consider the options of ground ambulance, air transport, and helicopter transport.
- Goal of triage is to get the person to the most appropriate level of care as quickly as possible.
- Triage nurse needs to have a broad range of knowledge and skills due to limited support and specialized backup.
- Triage needs may occur outside the hospital setting, that is, community health nurse, telephone triage nurse to avoid an unnecessary trip to the ED or facility.
- There may be a greater concern for personal safety due to violent patients, families, and visitors due to a lack of resources, police, additional security staff.

Legal Considerations

The triage nurse needs to be aware of the variety of legal constraints and requirements affecting triage practices.

- **Emergency Medical Treatment and Active Labor Act (EMTALA):** This act helps to protect patients from being transferred or refused care when unstable or in labor. It says that a patient must be stabilized before transferring to another facility. This is important for the triage nurse because once a patient presents to triage, he or she must be triaged and have a MSE to ensure his or her condition is stable before transfer or discharge. It also prohibits pregnant women from being transferred in active labor.

- **MSE** determines whether a person has an emergency medical condition, or if a woman is in active labor, and if so must medically stabilize or appropriately transfer to an appropriate level of care. Some facilities use advanced practice providers in this role at triage to help relieve congestion in the ED, improve wait times, and provide treatment as appropriate.
  - **MSE is not triage, but can be conducted in the triage environment** by a MD, NP, PA, or other qualified medical person. Providing a MSE in the triage environment must be approved by the governing body of the hospital or facility.
  - **MSE** or treatment should not be delayed to determine the person's ability to pay. Some EDs do not gather any information regarding insurance or ability to pay until after discharge instructions are completed to ensure compliance with this regulation.
  - **MSE components** should include the following to ensure that the individual is stable enough for transfer or redirecting to other healthcare services:
    - Chief complaint
    - Vital signs
    - Mental status
    - General appearance
    - Ability to ambulate
    - Focused physician/NP/PA examination
    - Results of examination must be documented
    - Assign acuity and categorize into degree of urgency
    - Document that the patient does not have an emergency medical condition and can be safely referred to other healthcare resources
- **Consents**
  - **Expressed Consent:** Person gives consent for treatment. If it is a verbal consent, documentation should reflect that verbal consent was given.
  - **Implied Consent:** Person is unable to give consent and there is a threat to life, limb, or vision such as in a trauma victim or when unconscious and requires intubation.
  - **Involuntary Consent:** Person is incompetent, refuses consent, and requires treatment. The level of competence is determined by the provider and treatment can be provided without the person's consent if determined by the provider that refusal to consent may result in a threat to life or limb. The person may be mentally impaired and a threat to themselves or others, and can be treated and held without their consent.
  - **Informed Consent:** Person is competent and gives consent for a specific procedure or service.

Maintaining Quality

Triage competency is the ability to apply knowledge and training to the triage process. The focus should always be patient safety. It is ongoing and helps to ensure staff accountability for making safe assessments, decision-making, and disposition decisions. Competency can be measured through direct observation of the nurse engaged in the triage process, chart review, and feedback from other nurses, providers, and patients. Triage competency should include evaluation of the following components:

- **Critical Thinking Skills:** Evaluate the nurse's ability to solve problems and make decisions. This can be measured through direct observation, feedback from other providers, or retrospective chart review. The ability to think critically is essential in the triage nursing process.
- **Technical Skills:** Evaluate the nurse's ability to apply principals of the triage process, document the assessment, use triage protocols/guidelines appropriately, and prioritize patient acuity. This can be measured through direct observation, retrospective chart review, and feedback from other providers and patients.
- **Interpersonal Skills:** Evaluate the nurse's ability to interact with patients, families, and other members of the care team. The first impression a patient may have of the ED experience begins with the triage nurse and the ability of the nurse to impart a sense of caring and competence. It is critical for the patient to have a positive experience. This can be measured through direct observation, feedback from other providers, patients, and families.

Ensuring and measuring quality is the responsibility of the whole care team and not just the manager or supervisor providing feedback through yearly performance reviews. It is an ongoing process of self-reflection and feedback from others. This can be accomplished in a number of ways.

- Use the Triage Skills Assessment form in Appendix F, Triage Assessment Skills Checklist, through direct observation or in scenario practice.
- Use the Chart Audit Tool in Appendix G, Chart Audit Tool, for retrospective chart review conducted by other nurses and the nurse who performed the triage. Engaging all the nurses in the review process helps to develop and enhance everyone's learning and development.
- Establish a list of key conditions and have each nurse focus on pulling five condition-specific cases each month to review and critique. These can be hospital quality indicators of ED-specific concerns such as chest pain, abdominal pain, pediatrics, mental health problems, stroke, and pneumonia.

- Assign a preceptor to all nurses new at triage.
- Provide both concurrent and retrospective chart reviews and provide feedback to the nurses to enhance their learning. See Chart Audit form in Appendix G, Chart Audit Tool.
- Involve staff members in any change process involving triage flow, system change, documentation to ensure compliance with the changes.
- Monitor patient complaints and poor outcomes related to triage decisions and process. Provide feedback. Follow up on all patient complaints.
- If nurse-initiated order sets or advance practice protocols are used, monitor their use and adherence to the protocols, policies, and procedures.
- Post information regarding current community outbreaks and any requirements for isolation.
- Regularly review triage policies and procedures for accuracy and consistency with current trends and practices. Ensure all staff are up to date with any changes to policies and procedures.
- Encourage continued learning and skill enhancement through educations, conferences, online resources, and webinars.

Training

Provide initial and ongoing training for all members of the team engaged in the triage process. This can be accomplished through one-to-one training, preceptors, group training, or a combination of all three approaches. This manual provides a variety of tools to assist in the training process.

- Review the **Preface** to gain better understanding of the 5-Tier Triage protocol components and their use in the triage process.
- Review current triage policies and procedures.
- If nurse-initiated order sets or advance practice protocols are used, review the order sets and policies for their use in triage.
- Review the **Training Exercises** (Appendix E, Triage Training Exercises) individually or in groups.
- Review **Key Questions** (Appendix B, Key Questions to Ask Triage Nurses) to gain a better understanding of condition-specific questions relevant to the triage process and decision-making.
- Review **Triage Pearls** to learn from the experience of others (Appendix C, Triage Pearls).
- Discuss ways to continually improve customer services. Have staff share successes and not-so-successful encounters for others to learn from those experiences.
- Conduct a scavenger hunt to locate supplies, backup paper charts, panic button, wheel chairs, waiting areas, observation area, EKG machine, and ice machine.
- Conduct triage training for all staff new to triage (see Appendix D, Triage Training Outline).

- Review Reference Charts in Appendices I to T to gain better understanding of additional information provided in this book to enhance nursing learning and knowledge base.
  - Differential Assessment of Abdominal Pain
  - Differential Assessment of Chest Pain
  - Headache: Common Characteristics
  - MVA Triage Questions
  - Mechanisms of Injury: Adult
  - Mechanisms of Injury: School Age and Adolescent (7–17 years old)
  - Mechanisms of Injury: Toddler and Preschooler (1–6 years old)
  - Mechanisms of Injury: Infant (birth to 1 year old)
  - Drugs of Abuse
  - Poisonings
  - Biological Agents/Chemical Agents
  - Communicable Diseases, Colds Versus Flu, and Sexually Transmitted Diseases

Managing Mass Casualties and Active Shooter Incidents

Mass casualty incidents (MCIs) can occur inside or outside the facility and have a major impact on the ED and the role of the triage nurse. To avoid overwhelming triage, an alternative triage site may need to be quickly established. A MCI can be related to dramatic weather, traumatic accidents, fires, exposures, pandemics, terrorist incidents, or active shooter incidents.

- ED may need to turn waiting areas into treatment areas.
- It is imperative that alternative triage sites be established before the incident occurs. Some EDs have large portable triage bags with essential supplies, forms, and necessary equipment to take to the alternative sites. Suggestions may include adjacent conference rooms, covered porticos, any space close enough to the ED to move patients quickly requiring immediate treatment but far enough away from the entrance to prevent a major onslaught of patients and visitors overwhelming the ED entrance, and potential new treatment areas. Warm weather areas can be used to establish triage outside near the ED.
- Arriving ambulances can be triaged to holding areas or directly to a treatment bed, if available.
- Special tents can be purchased that essentially serve as an alternative facility. These tents can be heated, and can be set up to have electricity and water. Operating suites, treatment areas, and triage area can be separated within the tents. Many of these alternative treatment tents are stored in a trailer near the ED. Staff are specially trained to set up these tents and utilities. Although these tents were initially established for homeland security issues and hazmat incidents, any major catastrophic event can

destroy the current medical infrastructure and require additional alternative treatment facilities.
- The triage nurse should be familiar with MCI management in the local region and what systems local Emergency Medical Services (EMS) use to · categorize patients and need for treatment.

START Method Triage: Simple Triage and Rapid Treatment

The START method of triage is used when resources are overwhelmed and takes about 30 seconds. The triage nurse does not initiate treatment except to reposition the airway or provide direction to others to control bleeding. See listing for bleeding control kits under "Prepare for and Manage Active Shooter Incidents" after this section. The START method evaluates respirations, perfusion, and mental status. The system uses color-coded tags to signify the category of the victim and alert caregivers who should be moved to a treatment area first, or is safe to remain waiting until the most critical have been taken for treatment. START categories include the following:

- Deceased (black tag)—the person is not breathing and does not improve with repositioning the airway.
- Immediate (red tag)—the person has serious injuries but is not at high risk for early death. He or she may be in shock from blood loss or a head injury. Respirations are greater than 30 per minute, radial pulse absent or capillary refill greater than 2 seconds, or person is unable to follow simple commands.
- Delayed (yellow tag)—the person has serious injuries but is not at high risk for early death. Frequently reassess and reprioritize as needed.
- Minor (green tag)—the person is considered the walking wounded with minor injuries that do not require immediate attention.
- Uninjured—the person does not require medical attention.

Prepare for and Manage Active Shooter Incidents

With the surge in active shooter incidents over the past several years, it is important for healthcare facilities to prepare for such incidents through prevention, response during, and immediately after the incident.

Prevention
- Require all staff, patients, and visitors to wear identification badges.
- Empower staff to report suspicious activity.
- Ensure that locked doors remain locked and secure.
- Change codes to keypads frequently.
- Provide training and drills that allow staff to practice what to do in the event of a shooting incident. Involve all staff including physicians, security, and outside agencies such as the police and EMS.

- Learn the signs of a potentially violent situation and ways to prevent the situation.
- Learn what to do to be safe when faced with an active shooter.
- Identify exits.
- Identify places to hide safely, if necessary.
- Be prepared to work with law enforcement during the incident.

Response During the Incident: "Run, Hide, Fight"

- Run away from the area/facility.
- Leave behind personal belongings except a cell phone, if able to retrieve quickly and poses no additional danger.
- Remember, healthcare workers can do the most good for the greatest number of people once law enforcement has subdued the threat of gunfire.
- Avoid escalators and elevators.
- Instruct others to follow you out and away from the building.
- Call 911 when safe to do so.
- If running is not a safe option, hide in an area with few to no windows and in an area that provides greater protection. Lock and barricade doors and windows. Pull blinds and darken the room. Silence cell phones, pagers, and other electronic devices.
- Fight if running and hiding are not safe options. Try to disrupt the shooter using blunt force objects such as tables, chairs, and fire extinguishers.

Response After the Incident

- The facility's MCI plan should be activated.
- Primary focus should be on hemorrhage control, which is key to saving lives.
  - Apply direct pressure with both hands until additional help arrives.
  - Apply pressure with a pressure dressing or bleeding control gauze, if available.
  - If unable to control the bleeding with direct pressure, apply a tourniquet to the extremity, if available and trained in its application. Apply 2 to 3 inches above the wound. If unable to control the bleeding, may apply a second tourniquet 2 to 4 inches above the first one. Use a commercial tourniquet with a self-locking mechanism once applied. Label the tourniquet with time of application. Do not loosen tourniquet until patient is safely in a care facility that can take definitive action, that is, surgery. Avoid using improvised tourniquets unless properly trained in the type of material to use and application. Tourniquets can be safely applied (if direct pressure ineffective in controlling the bleeding) for 2 hours before risk of tissue damage.

- Hemorrhage control supplies should be readily accessible. Some facilities secure hemorrhage control kits with fire extinguishers or automated external defibrillators. Kits may include gloves, chest seals, commercial tourniquets, bleeding control gauze, trauma bandages for packing wounds, marking pen for labeling with time applied, and instructions for tourniquet application. Kits should be sufficient to treat 20 people.
- Provide a debriefing and psychological first aid to assist responders in dealing with the traumatic stress and emotional distress after an event.

Key Questions to Ask Triage Nurses

Demographics

Name

Age (date of birth)

Gender identification (LGBTQ)

History

Allergies

Past medical/surgical history

Medications

Recent antibiotic use

Use/abuse of street drugs, prescription drugs, alcohol (amount, frequency)

When were substances last used

Previous reactions (bee, allergen, contrast media, etc.)

Tetanus immunization

Vaccine history (diphtheria and tetanus [dT], hepatitis B, infectious diseases, etc.)

Type of insect/animal/snake

Infectious disease

Mechanism of injury

Implanted devices such as automatic implantable cardioverter-defibrillator (AICD), pacemaker, left ventricular assist device (LVAD), coronary artery bypass graft (CABG), valve replacement, medication pumps.

Date of last menses

Recent use of antibiotics

Ingestion (toxic substance, foreign body, etc.)

Inhalation injury

Foreign body

Stents, rods, screws, artificial joints

Trauma: assault, self-inflicted, sport, vehicle

Use of safety equipment (helmet, wrist guards, etc.)

Birth history (for infant)

Birth control used

Possibility of pregnancy

Number of saturated pads or tampons per hour

Pregnancy history

Gestational age

Wound contamination

Number of wet diapers (infant)

Last consensual intercourse

Last suicide attempt

Violent behavior (of patient)

Symptoms

Onset

Description of pain (location, onset, intensity)

Description of injury/wound (burn, MVA)

Hallucinations

Confusion

Signs

Vital signs

Oximetry reading

Peak flow reading

Blood glucose level

Weight

Entrance and exit wounds

Neurovascular status of extremity

Facial droop

Extremity weakness

Slurred speech

Glasgow Coma Scale score

Description of rash, speed of development

Extremity weakness

Neuropathy

Others

Exposure (substance, weather, etc.)

Cause of trauma (physical, emotional, etc.)

International travel

Drinking from wells, streams, unpasteurized cider/milk, etc.

Association with others who are sick

Homeless

Visual acuity

Drainage or feeding tube history (when placed, is it functioning correctly)

Urinary catheter details (when inserted, drainage, tube care, etc.)

Concussion protocol

Triage Pearls

All Ages

- Remember FAST when evaluating for a possible stroke:
  - **F**—facial drooping or weak smile on one side of the face
    - Ask the person to smile.
  - **A**—arm/leg weakness on one side of the body
    - Ask the person to hold arms out in front shoulder high for 10 seconds.
  - **S**—speech slurred or difficult to understand
  - **T**—time is critical and person may need to be taken back immediately to CT scanner
    - Call 911 if in an outpatient setting.
- Be on the alert for signs of withdrawal from drugs or alcohol; rapid heartbeat, diaphoresis, fever, auditory or visual hallucinations, or delusion.
- Be on the alert for signs of systemic inflammatory response syndrome (SIRS): temperature >38.0°C or <36.0°C, HR >90 beats per minute, RR >20 breaths per minute.
- Consult with peers when unsure or situation seems complex, err on the side of over triage in the interest of patient safety.
- Survey your work area and have an exit plan in the event you encounter a patient or visitor who may become violent, hostile, or threatening in any manner.
- Ask if person served in the military, as he or she may have additional health benefits and services.
- Be mindful of how a transgender person addresses himself/herself.
  - If unsure, ask how the person would like to be addressed.
- Focus on time-sensitive conditions when door-to-treatment time is critical: stroke, acute myocardial infarction (AMI), SIRS, etc.
- Be alert if a visitor refuses to allow the patient to be alone with caregivers: consider domestic violence, human trafficking, elder abuse, etc.
- Determine the ability of a developmentally delayed patient—each person will have different abilities to answer questions, ambulate, cooperate with triage assessment, etc.
- The sickest patient being triaged may be the quietest. Stay calm when considering high anxiety patients and visitors—they will not always be the most acute.

- Separate high-risk patients from others (immunocompromised, agitated, rival gangs, etc.)
- Watch the waiting room carefully for potential conflicts, decompensating patients/visitors, etc.

Mental Health

- Remain calm when working with all patients, especially those who are agitated, under the influence of drugs/alcohol, manic, hostile, hallucinating, or any other type of behavioral concern (or who has a visitor with any of these).
- Note the patient's general appearance (well-groomed, disheveled), activity level (hyperactive, distant, solemn), affects (sad, happy), eye contact (avoid eye contact, staring, etc.), speech (rapid, clear, slurred, slow), thought content (hearing voices, delusional, hallucinating, oriented, insight, judgment).

Pediatric

- An altered mental status in a pediatric patient should alert the nurse to the potential for sepsis, blood glucose problems, seizure activity, or meningitis.
- A sleeping baby does not mean that neurologic status is okay.
- While listening to the parents, be sure to look at the child.
  - If the child is old enough, include the child in the conversation.
  - Allow the child to make simple choices, to gain his or her trust.
  - Perform painful or scary tasks last, or it will be difficult to gain the child's trust.
- While caring for the child, also care for the parent. (If the parent is anxious, the child will be anxious, too.)
- Consider abuse when the history does not make sense or there are conflicting histories.
- Bradycardia can indicate hypoxia until proved otherwise.
- Infants younger than 6 months old are obligate nose breathers. (Any nasal obstruction can produce respiratory distress.)
- Dehydration can happen quickly as a result of inadequate fluid intake or fluid loss.
- Infants have an unstable temperature-regulating mechanism (high body surface area to weight ratio) and quickly become hypothermic as a result of exposure.

Geriatric

- The elderly have decreased pain perception due to decreased peripheral nerve sensitivity.
- A hearing problem in the elderly can be misconstrued as confusion.
- A person with dementia or who is nonverbal may be unable to describe what happened or what hurts, so look for signs of injury.
- Altered mental status may be one of the first signs of an infection, dehydration, urinary or bowel problems, alcohol or drug withdrawal, or a stroke.
- Patients in this age group may be slower to communicate and may need additional time allowed for triage: the nurse should speak slowly, clearly, and loud enough to be heard.
- Maintain good eye contact when communicating with the patient to help determine if he or she understands what you are asking.
- Medication reconciliation is important in this age group as these patients may be taking many different medications.
- Many structural and functional changes occur in this age group such as **decrease** in the following: tissue elasticity, distensibility of blood vessels, strength of respiratory muscles, number of function neurons, visual acuity and speed of dark adaptation, gastrointestinal peristalsis, glomerular filtration rate, bone density, and compensatory mechanisms in general.

Obstetric Patients

- Owing to increased blood volume during pregnancy, clinical signs of shock may be delayed.
- Normal vital signs may change to accommodate the physiologic changes of pregnancy.
- The enlarged uterus may cause changes to or compression of the heart, ribs, or gastrointestinal, urinary, and/or musculoskeletal systems.

Triage Training Outline

I. **Overview**
1. Purpose of Triage
2. Rapid Triage
3. Comprehensive Triage
4. Customer Service Focus/Tips for Success
   - Patient
   - Family
   - Visitors
   - Police
   - EMS
   - Scripting to help with wait times and process
   - Establishing rapport with the caller
   - Dealing with difficult patients or poor historians
5. Roles and Responsibilities Personnel
   - RN
   - LPN/LVN
   - Technician
   - Registration
   - Advanced providers PA/NP
6. Legal Considerations
   - EMTALA: Emergency Medical Treatment and Active Labor Act
   - MSE: medical screening exam
   - HIPAA: Health Insurance Portability and Accountability Act
   - Consents
   - LWBS: left without being seen
   - AMA: against medical advice
7. Triage in Healthcare Today
   - Urban centers
   - Community health hospital/healthcare centers
   - Urgent care
   - Rural/remote health centers
   - Response to MCIs/disasters/active shooter events
   - Large events

II. **Operational Considerations**
1. Policy and Procedure Review
2. Triage Flow

- o Rapid triage
- o Comprehensive triage
- o Registration
- o Door to bed
- o Waiting areas (general, triage, urgent, laboratory/EKG/radiology)
3. Nurse-Initiated Orders/Advanced Triage Protocols (if approved by facility)
   - o Criteria for using protocols
   - o Review protocols
     - □ Laboratory values
     - □ Medications
     - □ X-ray studies/radiology/CT
     - □ EKG
4. Documentation
   - o Paper
   - o Electronic medical record (EMR)
   - o Downtime procedures
5. Reassessment Policies While Waiting
6. Communicable Disease Outbreaks

III. **Protocol Review and Practice**
1. Review Structure 5-Tier Triage Protocols
   - o Key questions
   - o Assessment questions
   - o Nursing actions/needed resources
   - o Assigning acuity/disposition
2. Review Most Common Conditions Requiring Emergent Dispositions
3. Review Key Questions (Appendix B)
4. Review Triage Pearls (Appendix C)
5. Form Triads to Practice With Scenarios (see Appendix E, Triage Training Exercises)
6. Design a Scavenger Hunt Unique to Your Facility to Identity Most Common Conditions/Protocols to Address Those Conditions, Location of Supplies, Wheelchairs, Panic Buttons, Safety Escape Route, Paper Charts for EMR Downtime.

IV. **Quality Improvement (QI) Process**
1. Review QI Process and Forms
2. Focused Condition Reviews
3. Peer Chart Reviews (see Chart Audit Tool, Appendix G)
4. Complaint-Based Reviews

V. **Role of Triage in Disasters and MCIs**
1. Most Common and Potential MCIs in Local Environment
2. EMS Start System
3. Facility Disaster Plan
4. Active Shooter Incidents
5. Debriefing After an Incident

VI. **Summary and Evaluation**

Triage Training Exercises

Identifying Appropriate Nursing Intervention at Triage

- Select 10 protocols that would require nursing interventions at triage based on your facility's guidelines and procedures.
- Indicate, in the space provided, the name of the protocol, page number, intervention(s), expected outcome, and name of facility guideline.

Example
Protocol: Chest Pain

Page Number _____

Intervention(s): Vital Signs, Pulse Oximetry, IV, EKG, Oxygen Saturation, Monitor, Low-Dose Aspirin, Notify Physician

Expected Outcome: Reduce discomfort, reduce damage to heart, rapidly identify potential lethal conditions, reduce time to reperfusion

Facility Guideline: Nursing Standing Orders

1. **Protocol:** _____

   Page Number _____

   Intervention(s): _____

   Expected Outcome: _____

   Name of Facility Guideline: _____

2. **Protocol:** _____

   Page Number _____

   Intervention(s): _____

   Expected Outcome: _____

   Name of Facility Guideline: _____

3. Protocol: _____

   Page Number _____

   Intervention(s): _____

   Expected Outcome: _____

   Name of Facility Guideline: _____

4. Protocol: _____

   Page Number _____

   Intervention(s): _____

   Expected Outcome: _____

   Name of Facility Guideline: _____

5. Protocol: _____

   Page Number _____

   Intervention(s): _____

   Expected Outcome: _____

   Name of Facility Guideline: _____

6. Protocol: _____

   Page Number _____

   Intervention(s): _____

   Expected Outcome: _____

   Name of Facility Guideline: _____

7. Protocol: _____

   Page Number _____

   Intervention(s): _____

   Expected Outcome: _____

   Name of Facility Guideline: _____

8. Protocol: _____

   Page Number _____

   Intervention(s): _____

   Expected Outcome: _____

   Name of Facility Guideline: _____

9. Protocol: _____

   Page Number _____

   Intervention(s): _____

   Expected Outcome: _____

   Name of Facility Guideline: _____

10. Protocol: _____

    Page Number _____

    Intervention(s): _____

    Expected Outcome: _____

    Name of Facility Guideline: _____

Name _____   Date Completed _____

Reviewed by _____   Date Reviewed _____

Identifying How Age and Chronic Illness Impact the Assignment of an Acuity Level and Risk for Waiting to Be Seen

- Select 10 different protocols that impact the acuity level based on age, medical condition, or chronic illness.
- Indicate, in the space provided, the name of the protocol, page number, condition that impacted the acuity level, acuity level, risk for waiting, nursing considerations for referral to treatment.
- Consider facility guidelines for appropriate waiting times for each category.

Example

Protocol: Chest Pain

Page Number _____

Condition Impacting Acuity: Age >35 years and heart palpitations; recent trauma, childbirth, surgery, or history of blood clotting problems; history of diabetes; congestive heart failure or blood clotting problems

Acuity Level: Level 2

Risk for Waiting: High risk

Nursing Considerations: Emergent, refer for treatment within minutes.

1. **Protocol:** _____

   Page Number _____

   Condition Impacting Acuity: _____

   Acuity Level: _____

   Risk for Waiting: _____

   Nursing Consideration: _____

2. **Protocol:** _____

   Page Number _____

   Condition Impacting Acuity: _____

   Acuity Level: _____

   Risk for Waiting: _____

   Nursing Consideration: _____

3. **Protocol:** _____

   Page Number _____

   Condition Impacting Acuity: _____

   Acuity Level: _____

   Risk for Waiting: _____

   Nursing Consideration: _____

4. **Protocol:** _____

   Page Number _____

   Condition Impacting Acuity: _____

Acuity Level: _____

Risk for Waiting: _____

Nursing Consideration: _____

5. Protocol: _____

   Page Number _____

   Condition Impacting Acuity: _____

   Acuity Level: _____

   Risk for Waiting: _____

   Nursing Consideration: _____

6. Protocol: _____

   Page Number _____

   Condition Impacting Acuity: _____

   Acuity Level: _____

   Risk for Waiting: _____

   Nursing Consideration: _____

7. Protocol: _____

   Page Number _____

   Condition Impacting Acuity: _____

   Acuity Level: _____

   Risk for Waiting: _____

   Nursing Consideration: _____

8. Protocol: _____

   Page Number _____

   Condition Impacting Acuity: _____

   Acuity Level: _____

   Risk for Waiting: _____

   Nursing Consideration: _____

9. **Protocol:** _____

   Page Number _____

   Condition Impacting Acuity: _____

   Acuity Level: _____

   Risk for Waiting: _____

   Nursing Consideration: _____

10. **Protocol:** _____

    Page Number _____

    Condition Impacting Acuity: _____

    Acuity Level: _____

    Risk for Waiting: _____

    Nursing Consideration: _____

Name _____   **Date Completed** _____

Reviewed by _____   **Date Reviewed** _____

Scenario Practice

The purpose of this exercise is to help the nurse orient to the triage protocols and teach new nurses to recognize an emergent situation, appropriate disposition, and what to anticipate in terms of utilization of resources. In addition, it can assist the nurse to identify when it is appropriate to initiate diagnostic studies and interventions based on facility guidelines.

For each scenario described below, identify in the space provided the following:

- The acuity level and triage category based on the 5-tier triage system
- Time frame to be seen by the physician (consider facility policy for semi-urgent and nonurgent patients)
- Anticipated nursing considerations, interventions, medical diagnostics, procedures, and consultations
- The protocol used and associated page number

Example

A 58-year-old male has a chief complaint of midsternal chest pain, nausea, and diaphoresis for the past 2 hours. He describes his pain as 8/10 on the pain scale. His vital signs are BP 140/90, P 96, R 22.

Acuity Level: 2, High risk

Triage Category: Emergent

Time Frame to Be Seen: Should not wait to be seen

Nursing Considerations: Anticipate IV, laboratory values, EKG, monitor, medications, oxygen saturation

Protocol Referenced: Chest pain

Page Number _____

Scenarios

1. A 26-year-old woman has a chief complaint of urinary frequency and burning when she urinates. She denies flank pain or vaginal discharge. Her last menstrual period was 2 weeks ago. She is taking birth control pills. Her vital signs are BP 118/72, P 70, R 18, T 97.6°F.

   Acuity Level: _____ Triage Category: _____

   Time Frame to Be Seen: _____

   Nursing Considerations: _____

   Protocol Referenced: _____ Page Number _____

2. A 17-year-old man has a chief complaint of a sore throat since yesterday. He denies swollen or tender nodes or exudate in the back of the throat. He is able to swallow and handle his secretions well and speak in full sentences. He describes his pain as 5/10 on the pain scale. His vital signs are BP 114/76, P 70, R 18, T 98.6°F.

   Acuity Level: _____ Triage Category: _____

   Time Frame to Be Seen: _____

   Nursing Considerations: _____

   Protocol Referenced: _____ Page Number _____

3. A 19-year-old man has a chief complaint of nausea since this morning. He states he "threw up" once this morning. He denies diarrhea or abdominal pain. He has been able to tolerate fluids. His vital signs are BP 120/76, P 80, R 18, T 98.4°F.

   Acuity Level: _____ Triage Category: _____

   Time Frame to Be Seen: _____

Nursing Considerations: _____

Protocol Referenced: _____ Page Number _____

4. A 42-year-old woman has a chief complaint of a severe headache, described as the "worst headache of my life," that started 1 hour prior to
arrival. She describes her pain as 10/10 on the pain scale. She is awake
and alert, but obviously uncomfortable. She denies a head injury or history of headaches. Her vital signs are BP 150/80, P 90, R 20, T 98.2°F.

Acuity Level: _____ Triage Category: _____

Time Frame to Be Seen: _____

Nursing Considerations: _____

Protocol Referenced: _____ Page Number _____

5. A 68-year-old man reportedly collapsed at the mall and has been brought
in by the paramedics. His wife states that he had been complaining about
chest discomfort before collapsing. He was defibrillated three times and
CPR has been in progress for the past 20 minutes. His pupils remain
reactive to light.

Acuity Level: _____ Triage Category: _____

Time Frame to Be Seen: _____

Nursing Considerations: _____

Protocol Referenced: _____ Page Number _____

6. A 24-year-old man injured his ankle while playing basketball 2 hours
ago. He reportedly came down on his ankle and felt a pop. The ankle
is now painful, swollen, and ecchymotic. He states that he is unable to
bear weight on that extremity because of the discomfort. He describes
the pain as 6/10 on the pain scale. His vital signs are BP 110/60, P 80,
R 20, T 98.2°F.

Acuity Level: _____ Triage Category: _____

Time Frame to Be Seen: _____

Nursing Considerations: _____

Protocol Referenced: _____ Page Number _____

7. A 24-year-old woman has a chief complaint of dizziness and states her mind "feels fuzzy, she can't think straight." She states she has a history of diabetes and took her insulin this morning but cannot remember whether she ate breakfast or not. Her vital signs are BP 118/70, P 70, R 16, T 98.2°F.

Acuity Level: _____ Triage Category: _____

Time Frame to Be Seen: _____

Nursing Considerations: _____

Protocol Referenced: _____ Page Number _____

8. An 82-year-old woman has a chief complaint of "weakness, a little confused, and has no appetite." Her daughter states that she has generally been healthy and active up until the past few days. She also states that her mother had been complaining of "some burning with urination." Her vital signs are BP 118/70, P 80, R 18, T 100.6°F.

Acuity Level: _____ Triage Category: _____

Time Frame to Be Seen: _____

Nursing Considerations: _____

Protocol Referenced: _____ Page Number _____

9. A 19-year-old man has a chief complaint that he was stabbed in the chest twice by his girlfriend about 30 minutes ago. He states he is having some difficulty catching his breath. He is pale and his vital signs are BP 70/40, P 128, R 26, T 98.1°F.

Acuity Level: _____ Triage Category: _____

Time Frame to Be Seen: _____

Nursing Considerations: _____

Protocol Referenced: _____ Page Number _____

10. A 67-year-old man has a chief complaint of sudden weakness on his left side. He has a noticeable facial droop and is unsteady on his feet. He states that the symptoms started about 1 hour prior to arrival. His vital signs are BP 160/94, P 98, R 20, T 100.1°F.

Acuity Level: _____ Triage Category: _____

Time Frame to Be Seen: _____

Nursing Considerations: _____

Protocol Referenced: _____ Page Number _____

11. A 17-year-old man has a chief complaint of left ear pain since last night. He states this happens every time he goes swimming, but this time he cannot seem to shake it. His vital signs are BP 116/72, P 74, R 16, T 98.2°F.

Acuity Level: _____ Triage Category: _____

Time Frame to Be Seen: _____

Nursing Considerations: _____

Protocol Referenced: _____ Page Number _____

12. A 33-year-old man has a chief complaint of nausea, vomiting, and diarrhea for 3 days. He states that he has been ill since returning from a camping trip a few days ago. He has been unable to keep anything down and nothing has worked to stop the vomiting or diarrhea. His vital signs are BP 106/62, P 88, R 18, T 98.4°F.

Acuity Level: _____ Triage Category: _____

Time Frame to Be Seen: _____

Nursing Considerations: _____

Protocol Referenced: _____ Page Number _____

13. A 72-year-old man has a chief complaint of abdominal pain. He states it is "pretty bad" and radiates into his back. His wife states that the pain started about 2 hours ago and he nearly fainted several times prior to arrival in the ED. His vital signs are BP 174/92, P 88, R 20, T 98.2°F. Pain scale rating: 7/10.

Acuity Level: _____ Triage Category: _____

Time Frame to Be Seen: _____

Nursing Considerations: _____

Protocol Referenced: _____ Page Number _____

14. A 42-year-old man is concerned he may have an allergic reaction to something he ate. He recently ingested some peanut oil by accident and states he has had a severe allergy to peanuts in the past. His vital signs are BP 144/88, P 108, R 24, T 98.2°F. He suddenly collapses after you take his vital signs.

Acuity Level: _____ Triage Category: _____

Time Frame to Be Seen: _____

Nursing Considerations: _____

Protocol Referenced: _____ Page Number _____

15. A 48-year-old man has a chief complaint of vomiting blood and abdominal pain. He is pale and diaphoretic. His vital signs are BP 80/50, P 118, R 24, T 98.2°F. Pain scale rating: 6/10.

Acuity Level: _____ Triage Category: _____

Time Frame to Be Seen: _____

Nursing Considerations: _____

Protocol Referenced: _____ Page Number _____

16. A 17-year-old woman has a chief complaint of dental pain. She has a history of right upper molar pain and swelling for the past 10 days. She states she has been unable to get in to see a dentist for the past 2 weeks. She is alert, oriented, and breathing without difficulty. Her vital signs are BP 126/70, P 68, R 18, T 98.4°F. Pain scale rating: 6/10.

Acuity Level: _____ Triage Category: _____

Time Frame to Be Seen: _____

Nursing Considerations: _____

Protocol Referenced: _____ Page Number _____

17. A 28-year-old woman has a chief complaint of a headache, rated 7/10 on the pain scale. She has nausea and photophobia. She states that this episode is similar to other migraines she has experienced in the past, but this one has not responded to her usual homecare measures and pain medications. Her vital signs are BP 118/68, P 88, R 22, T 98.2°F.

Acuity Level: _____ Triage Category: _____

Time Frame to Be Seen: _____

Nursing Considerations: _____

Protocol Referenced: _____ Page Number _____

18. A 34-year-old woman has a chief complaint of facial injuries, including ecchymosis to both eyes, a swollen lip, and dried blood around the nose. She states a book fell off the shelf and hit her in the face. Her vital signs are BP 138/78, P 88, R 22, T 98.2°F. Pain scale rating: 5/10.

Acuity Level: _____ Triage Category: _____

Time Frame to Be Seen: _____

Nursing Considerations: _____

Protocol Referenced: _____ Page Number _____

19. A 77-year-old woman has a chief complaint of a shoulder injury. She states she tripped and fell about 3 hours ago on her right shoulder. She is able to ambulate and has pain and swelling to the right upper arm. She has limited range of motion in the right arm. Her circulation, sensation, and movement are intact. Her vital signs are BP 138/78, P 88, R 20, T 98.2°F. Pain scale rating: 7/10.

Acuity Level: _____ Triage Category: _____

Time Frame to Be Seen: _____

Nursing Considerations: _____

Protocol Referenced: _____ Page Number _____

20. A 28-year-old man has a chief complaint of splashing cleaning fluid in both eyes 20 minutes ago. He tried to splash cold water into his eyes immediately afterward. His eyes are reddened, swollen, and painful. He rates his pain 7/10 on the pain scale. His vital signs are BP 128/78, P 88, R 20, T 98.2°F.

Acuity Level: _____ Triage Category: _____

Time Frame to Be Seen: _____

Nursing Considerations: _____

Protocol Referenced: _____ Page Number _____

Triage Assessment Skills Checklist

	TIME: _____			TIME: _____		
	Yes	No	N/A	Yes	No	N/A
Greeting						
• Greets patient courteously						
• Utilizes proper opening script (identifies self and patient)						
• Gathers appropriate demographic data						
• Comments:						
Assessment						
• Identifies emergency signs and symptoms						
• Measures vital signs (per facility guidelines)						
• Gathers appropriate patient history						
• Upgrades patient to higher level of urgency as needed (child, confused adult, foreign-language speaker, etc.)						
• Makes assignment for care and acuity within appropriate time frame						
• Performs medication reconciliation per facility guidelines						
• Orders appropriate medications or diagnostic studies per facility protocol						

(continued)

	Yes	No	N/A	Yes	No	N/A
• Offers and documents interim care measures if not emergency (splint, ice pack, emesis basin, etc.)						
• Documents appropriate, including assessment, nursing interventions, acuity, and disposition						
• Comments:						
Communication Skills						
• Conveys a positive image of organization						
• Maintains a courteous, calm, professional demeanor						
• Exhibits ability to adapt to different personalities, emotions, and behaviors						
• Assumes control of the interview: listens attentively, interjects appropriately, and elicits necessary information						
• Takes time with the patient when appropriate; efficient without compromising quality						
• Uses simple, direct language that the patient understands						
• Does not interrupt the patient/parent/visitor						
• Speaks at a moderate rate with expressive modulation of tone						
• Comments:						
Closing						
• Ends interview efficiently						
• Informs patient of next step and expected wait						

(continued)

	Yes	No	N/A	Yes	No	N/A
• If patient has to wait, instructs patient/family member to inform triage nurse of any changes or worsening of the problem while waiting						
• Comments:						

RN Name: _____ Preceptor/reviewer: _____ Date: _____

Chart Audit Tool

Name of Triage Nurse: _____   Date and Time of Triage: _____

Name of Reviewer: _____   Date of Review: _____

INDICATOR	YES	NO	N/A
Date and time of patient arrival			
Time of triage			
Chief complaint			
Date/time of onset of symptoms			
Allergies			
Prior medical/surgical history			
Severity of symptoms (pain scale if pain present)			
Medications			
Vital signs			
Treatment prior to arrival			
Key questions addressed relevant to chief complaint (i.e., implanted device, additional symptoms, recent travel, number of pads, diapers, oxygen saturation; see Appendix B, Key Questions to Ask Triage Nurses, for list of key questions)			
Acuity assigned			
Disposition: registration, treatment room, waiting room, triage waiting area, radiology, OB, LWBS, AMA, police			
Nurse-initiated orders/advanced triage protocols			
Signature of triage nurse			

Comments: _____

_____

Date and time audit feedback provided to triage nurse: _____

_____

Triage Log

ARRIVAL DATE TIME	PATIENT NAME, AGE, GENDER	SYMPTOM CONCERN ONSET	ACUITY ASSIGNMENT	DISPOSITION	NURSE NAME	COMMENTS TREAT-MENTS

Differential Assessment of Abdominal Pain

POSSIBLE DIAGNOSIS	SIGNS AND SYMPTOMS
Abdominal aortic aneurysm	Asymptomatic until leakage or rupture occurs Abrupt onset of severe back, flank, or abdominal pain Pulsatile abdominal mass, mottling of lower extremities, signs of shock
Appendicitis	Diffuse pain in epigastric or periumbilical area for 1–2 days Localization of pain over the right lower quadrant between the umbilicus and right iliac crest Anorexia, nausea/vomiting, fever, tachycardia, pallor, peritoneal signs Increased pain with stairs, walking, etc.
Bowel obstruction	Severe, crampy, colicky abdominal pain Vomiting, constipation, hypotension, tachycardia, abdominal distention, hyperactive bowel sounds, fever
Cholecystitis (inflammation of gallbladder)	Colicky discomfort in the right upper quadrant midepigastric area Pain radiating to the shoulders and back Nausea/vomiting, fever, tachycardia, tachypnea, abdominal guarding, jaundice, malaise
Cholelithiasis (presence of gallbladder stones)	Severe, steady, or colicky pain in the upper abdominal quadrant, often right-sided Pain usually begins 3–6 hours after a large meal Pain radiation to scapula, back, or right shoulder Nausea, vomiting, dyspepsia, mild to moderate jaundice
Constipation/fecal impaction	Clinically defined as defecation <3 times per week Each patient may interpret the symptoms differently Fatigue, abdominal discomfort, headache, low back pain, anorexia, restlessness
Duodenal or ileojejunal hematoma	Caused by a blow to the abdomen Immediate bruising over upper quadrant of abdomen
Epididymitis	Infection or inflammation of the epididymis Swelling and enlargement of the epididymis, sudden swelling of the spermatic cord, fever, dysuria, urethral discharge

(continued)

POSSIBLE DIAGNOSIS	SIGNS AND SYMPTOMS
Intussusception	Paroxysms of acute abdominal pain, intermittent with pain-free episodes Currant jelly, mucus-type stools or rectal bleeding Fever, lethargy, vomiting (food, mucus, fecal matter), dehydration
Orchitis	Inflammation or infection of the testicle Intense pain and swelling of the scrotum, dysuria, urethral discharge, fever, discomfort in the groin/lower abdomen, acute illness
Pancreatitis	Severe, constant, upper quadrant midepigastric pain that radiates to the midback Pain worsens when lying flat on back, relieved when lying on side with knees drawn up Nausea, vomiting, fever, pallor, hypotension, tachycardia, tachypnea, restlessness, malaise, fatty or foul-smelling stools, abdominal distention, pulmonary crackles
Peritonitis	Severe pain that gradually increases in intensity and worsens with movement Riding in car, climbing stairs, or jumping on one foot greatly worsens pain Radiation of pain to shoulder, back, or chest Nausea, vomiting, fever, abdominal distention, rigidity, and tenderness
Renal calculi	Location of stone depicts associated pain: flank, lower abdominal quadrant, low back, groin, testicular, labial, or urethral meatus Pain radiation varies on stone location Nausea, vomiting, pallor, diaphoresis, marked restlessness, dehydration
Ruptured ovarian cyst	Sudden, severe, unilateral lower quadrant abdominal pain associated with exercise or intercourse Delayed or prolonged menstruation, vomiting, ascites, signs of peritonitis
Tubal pregnancy	Intermittent diffuse abdominal pain Radiation of pain to shoulder Vaginal spotting/bleeding, syncope, dizziness, signs of peritonitis or shock
Urinary tract infection	Lower quadrant abdominal or pelvic pain Urinary burning, frequency, urgency, hematuria, foul-smelling urine, fever, bladder spasms
• Cystitis	Dysuria, frequency/urgency, fever, hematuria
• Pyelonephritis	Flank or back pain Urinary frequency, dysuria, fever, malaise, nausea, vomiting, chills

(continued)

POSSIBLE DIAGNOSIS	SIGNS AND SYMPTOMS
• Prostatitis	Perineal aching, low back pain, frequency, dysuria, fever, malaise, urethral discharge, prostate swelling
Testicular torsion	Sudden onset of severe, unilateral testicular pain and tenderness Nausea, vomiting, fever, scrotal mass
Ulcer (gastric, duodenal, esophageal)	Colicky, burning, squeezing pain in the epigastric or midback area Pain intensity is variable, often begins 1–3 hours after meals, worsens at night Nausea, vomiting, hematemesis, abdominal guarding, decreased or absent bowel sounds

Differential Assessment of Chest Pain

SYSTEM	CAUSE	CHARACTERISTICS
Cardiovascular	Acute myocardial infarction	Pain may be described as aching, pressing, squeezing, burning, tightness. Intensity: vague to severe Location of pain may be substernal, epigastric, or between the shoulder blades Pain may radiate to the neck, jaw, arm, back Women may describe symptoms more of nausea, fatigue, shortness of breath Diabetic neuropathy patients may have only vague pain
	Aneurysm	Pain may be described as searing, continuous, severe Pain may radiate to the back, neck, or shoulder(s) Associated signs and symptoms: hypotension, diaphoresis, syncope
	Angina	Pain may be described as squeezing, pressing, tight, relieved with rest or nitroglycerin Pain may be persistent and intermittent Occurs with activity, anxiety, sex, heavy meals, smoking, or at rest Associated signs and symptoms: dyspnea, nausea, vomiting, diaphoresis, indigestion
	Cardiac contusion	Cardiac compression between the sternum and vertebral column (falls, MVAs, blunt chest trauma, etc.) Assess for crush injury to the chest with traumatic falls from skiing, skateboarding, motocross, or other extreme sports May have EKG changes such as right bundle branch block, ST-T wave abnormalities, Q waves, atrial fibrillation, premature ventricular contractions, and A-V conduction disturbances

(continued)

SYSTEM	CAUSE	CHARACTERISTICS
Cardiovascular (cont.)	Heart transplant	*Rejection* may present with low-grade fever, fatigue, dyspnea, peripheral edema, pulmonary crackles, malaise, pericardial friction rub, arrhythmias, decreased EKG voltage, hypotension, increased jugular distention
		Infection may be masked by use of immuno-suppressive therapy; look for low-grade fever, cough, and malaise *Coronary heart disease* is common in patients with heart transplants
	Pericarditis	Pain may be described as severe, continuous, worse when lying on left side Radiation of pain to shoulder or neck History may include recent cardiac surgery, viral illness, or myocardial infarction Diffuse ST segment elevation in multiple leads PQ segment depression
	Tachydys-rhythmia	Pain may be described as severe, crushing, or generalized over chest Associated signs and symptoms: anxiety, tachycardia, dizziness, impending doom
Gastrointestinal	Hiatal hernia	Pain may be described as sharp, over the epigastrium Occurs with heavy meals, bending over, lying down
	Gastroesopha-geal reflux disease	Pain may be described as burning, heartburn, pressing Nonradiating pain, not influenced by activity
Musculoskeletal	Costochondritis	Pain may be described as sharp or severe Localized to affected area with tenderness on palpation Associated signs and symptoms: cough, "cold"
	Muscle strain	Pain may be described as aching Occurs with increased use or exercise of upper-body muscles Pain is severe, with localization over area of trauma Pain worsens with palpations, movement, or cough May have dyspnea

(continued)

SYSTEM	CAUSE	CHARACTERISTICS
Pulmonary	Noxious fumes/ smoke inhalation	Pain may be described as searing; sense of suffocation History includes exposure to fire, pesticide, carbon monoxide, paint, chemicals Associated signs and symptoms: dyspnea, hypoxia, cough, pallor, ashen skin, cyanosis, singed nasal hairs, soot in oropharynx, gray or black sputum, hoarseness, drooling Those with carbon monoxide poisoning may additionally show nausea, headache, confusion, dizziness, irritability, decreased judgment, ataxia, collapse
	Pleural effusion	Pain may be described as sharp, localized, gradual onset, yet continuous Dyspnea on exertion or at rest Pain worsens with breathing, coughing, movement Common in smokers
	Pneumonia	Pain may be described as continuous, dull discomfort to severe pain Associated signs and symptoms: fever, shortness of breath, tachycardia, malaise, cough, tachypnea Children may complain of abdominal pain instead of chest pain
	Pneumothorax	Pain may be described as sudden onset, sharp, severe Associated signs and symptoms: shortness of breath
	Pulmonary embolism	Acute shortness of breath Risk factors include recent long bone fractures, surgery, smoking, use of oral contraceptives, sitting for long periods of time (e.g., long air travel)
Other	Anxiety	Pain may be described as aching, stabbing Associated with stressful event, anxiety Associated signs and symptoms: hyperventilation, carpal spasms, palpitations, weakness, fear, sense of impending doom

A-V, atrioventricular; MVA, motor vehicle accident.

Source: Reproduced with permission from Grossman, V. (2003). *Quick reference to triage* (2nd ed.). Philadelphia, PA: Lippincott Williams & Wilkins.

Headache: Common Characteristics

HEADACHE TYPE	CHARACTERISTICS

Cerebellar hemorrhage	Pain:
	    Moderate to severe
	Associated signs and symptoms:
	    Confusion
	    Vomiting
	    Altered gait

Cluster headaches	Pain:
	    Very painful
	    Knifelike
	    Unilateral
	    Over the eye
	Associated signs and symptoms:
	    Excessive tearing
	    Facial swelling
	    Redness of the eye
	    Diaphoresis

Increased intracranial pressure	Pain:
	    Usually not excruciating
	Associated symptoms:
	    Nausea or vomiting
	    Lethargy
	    Diplopia
	    Transient visual difficulty

Meningitis	Pain:
	    Mild to severe
	    Neck pain or stiffness
	Associated signs and symptoms:
	    Fever
	    Malaise
	    Decreased appetite
	    Irritability

(continued)

HEADACHE TYPE	CHARACTERISTICS

Migraines	Pain:
	    Periodic with gradual onset
	    Throbbing, severe
	    Frequently unilateral, may progress to bilateral
	    Often above the eye(s)
	Associated signs and symptoms:
	    Photophobia
	    Sensitivity to sound
	    Nausea
	    Vomiting

Sinus headache	Pain:
	    Over the sinus areas (above the eyes, beside the nose, or over the cheekbone)
	Associated signs and symptoms:
	    Fever
	    Nasal drainage or congestion
	    Ear pain
	    Tenderness, swelling, or erythema of the sinus area

Subarachnoid hemorrhage	Pain:
	    "Worst headache of my life"
	Associated signs and symptoms:
	    With or without transient impairment of consciousness

Tension	Pain:
	    Diffuse yet steady dull pain or pressure
	    "Band-like" (back of head and neck, across forehead, and/or temporal areas)

MVA Triage Questions

When did the accident occur?

- Day
- Time

Where did it occur?

- Highway
- Country road
- City street
- Off road
- Racetrack

Was the patient wearing a seat belt?

- What type? (Lap, shoulder, etc.)
- Effectiveness during the accident

What speed was the patient's car traveling?

- Approximate speed of other vehicles involved in accident
- Approximate speed of patient's vehicle

Where was the patient sitting in the car?

- Driver
- Front-seat passenger
- Back-seat passenger
- Box of the truck

What kind of vehicle was the patient in? What damage was done to the vehicle?

- Sport utility vehicle
- Compact car
- Other motorized vehicle
- Motorcycle

Did the airbag deploy?

- Which airbag deployed? (Front, side, etc.)

Did the patient lose consciousness?

- For how long?

What is the last thing the patient remembers *before* the accident? What is the first thing the patient remembers *after* the accident? How was the patient injured in the car?

- Flying objects within the car
- Car crushed by other vehicle, tree, pole, etc.

Was the patient thrown from the car?

- Was something in the car thrown against the patient?

Was the patient ambulatory at the scene?

- Did the patient need to be extricated from the vehicle?
- How long did it take?

Were there any other people in the car?

- Were they injured?
- What are their injuries?

Was the pediatric patient in a car seat?

- Where was the car seat located within the vehicle?
- Was it struck by a deployed air bag?
- Was the car seat strapped tightly with the seat belt?

Were there law enforcement personnel at the scene?

- If so, which agency?

Does the patient wear

- Contact lenses?
- Glasses?
- Hearing aid?
- Were they worn at the scene?

- Dentures?
- Female patients: Is a tampon in place?
- Insulin pump? Pacemaker? Internal cardiac defibrillator? Other medical device?

Where is the patient experiencing pain?

Is the patient taking any medication, especially aspirin or other anticoagulants?

Is there anyone the patient wishes to have notified?

Mechanisms of Injury: Adult

TRAUMA	ASSOCIATED INJURIES
Pedestrian struck by car • Adult point of impact is usually knee/hip	Fractures of the femur, tibia, and fibula on side of impact Fractured pelvis Contralateral ligament damage to knee
Pedestrian struck by car • Short adult/child point of impact involves chest and/or head	Contralateral skull fracture Chest injury with rib and/or sternal fracture May be thrown, resulting in head/back injury Shoulder dislocation and/or scapular fracture Patellar and lower femur fracture
Pedestrian dragged under a vehicle	Pelvic fracture
MVA: Unrestrained front-seat passenger • Front impact	Posterior dislocation of acetabulum Fractures of femurs and/or patellas
MVA: Unrestrained driver • Front impact	Head injury, C-spine injury, pelvic fracture Flail chest, fractured sternum Aortic or tracheal tears Pulmonary/cardiac contusion Ruptured or lacerated liver or spleen Femur and/or patellar fracture, hip dislocation
MVA: Unrestrained driver or passenger • Side impact	Chest: flail, fractured sternum, pulmonary/cardiac contusion Fractures of clavicle, acetabulum, pelvis Lateral neck strain or injury Driver: ruptured spleen Passenger: ruptured liver
MVA: Passenger without headrest restraint • Rear impact	Hyperextension of neck resulting in high C-spine or vertebral fracture or ruptured disc(s), causing epidural hemorrhage, edema, spinal cord compression

(continued)

TRAUMA	ASSOCIATED INJURIES
MVA: Rotational force from spinning car	Combination of frontal and side impact-induced injuries
MVA: Rollover of vehicle	Multitude of external and internal injuries
MVA: Ejection from vehicle	Injuries at point of impact
MVA: Restrained driver or passenger	Compression of soft tissue organs, C-spine injuries, rib and sternal fractures, cardiac contusions, ruptured diaphragm Lap belt only: head, neck, facial, and chest injuries Shoulder strap only: severe neck injury, decapitation Air bag deployed: facial injuries, abrasions/burns of arms
Fall • Landing on feet • Landing on buttocks	Compression fractures of lumbosacral spine Fractures of calcaneus Compression fracture of lumbar vertebrae Pelvic fracture Coccyx fracture
Diving • Head first	Forceful cervical spine compression resulting in fracture, dislocation, and/or displacement of vertebral bone fragments into spinal canal
Blunt head trauma • Person's moving head strikes a stationary object	Coup/contra-coup injury Depressed skull fracture Cerebral hematoma, contusions, or laceration
Blunt chest trauma • Moving object strikes a person's chest	Pulmonary contusion Hemothorax Rib fractures
Crush injury to chest	Traumatic asphyxia • Assess for crush injuries to the chest with traumatic falls from skiing, skateboarding, motocross, and other extreme sports • Crushing trauma forces blood from heart via the superior vena cava to veins of the head, neck, and upper chest, causing subconjunctival and/or retinal hemorrhage, conjunctival edema, and characteristic deep violet skin color

MVA, motor vehicle accident.

APPENDIX N

Mechanisms of Injury: School Age and Adolescent (7–17 years old)

Emergency Nursing Triage for Mechanisms of Injury: School Age and Adolescent Children

TRAUMA	ASSOCIATED INJURIES
Assaults	Head/chest/abdomen: closed or open injuries, fractures, C-spine injury, lacerations, organ trauma
Bicycle-related injuries	Head: closed or open injuries Chest: pulmonary/cardiac contusion, pneumothorax, rib fractures
Burns (flames, explosions, chemical)	Surface trauma; risk of multiple trauma exists
Drowning	Respiratory: acute respiratory distress syndrome
Falls	Head: cerebral swelling, epidural/subdural hematoma, skull fracture, C-spine injury Chest: pulmonary/cardiac contusion, hemothorax/pneumothorax Abdomen, skeletal, etc.: same as for MVAs
Farm injuries	Crush injuries
Minor trauma (superficial lacerations)	Surface trauma: lacerations, contusions
MVAs (occupant, pedestrian)	Head: cerebral swelling, epidural/subdural hematoma, skull fractures, C-spine injuries Chest: pulmonary/cardiac contusion, hemothorax or pneumothorax rib fractures Abdomen: • Liver: fracture, laceration • Spleen: hematoma, laceration, rupture • Kidney: hematoma, contusion, hematuria • Pancreas: contusion Miscellaneous: surface trauma, bony fractures
Penetrating trauma (stabbing, gunshot wounds)	Head/chest/abdomen: variety of injuries to internal organs

(continued)

TRAUMA	ASSOCIATED INJURIES
Sports-related injuries	Head: C-spine injuries, concussion Chest: rib fractures, pulmonary/cardiac contusions Abdomen: same as MVA possibilities
Suicide (ingestion, gunshot, hanging)	Head: C-spine injury from hanging Chest/abdomen: variety of injuries from penetrating trauma, falls, MVAs

MVA, motor vehicle accident.

Mechanisms of Injury: Toddler and Preschooler (1-6 years old)

Emergency Nursing Triage for Mechanisms of Injury: Toddler and Preschooler

Common Mechanisms of Injury

- Motor vehicle–related injuries
  - Occupant
  - Pedestrian
  - Bicycle
- Burns
  - Scald and flame
- Drownings
- Ingestions
- Minor surface trauma
- Child abuse
- Firearms (preschoolers)
- Falls
- Sledding
- Choking
- Animal bites
- Sports

INJURY PATTERN	RISK FACTORS	ASSOCIATED INJURIES
Abdomen	Pliable pelvic girdle fails to protect internal organs Proportionately larger abdominal organs Ribs do not protect upper abdominal contents Organs are in close proximity to each other Portion of bowel adheres to spine	Laceration, fracture, hematoma to solid organs (liver, spleen, kidney): MVAs, falls, abuse Hematoma to hollow organs: (esophagus, stomach, intestines): MVAs

(continued)

INJURY PATTERN	RISK FACTORS	ASSOCIATED INJURIES
Chest	Short trachea Compliant chest wall Mobile mediastinal structures Major vessels lack valves and predispose to traumatic asphyxia	Pulmonary/cardiac contusions: MVAs, falls, sledding Pneumothorax: MVAs, falls, abuse Traumatic asphyxia: MVAs
Head	Thin, pliable bony structures predispose to diffuse cerebral injuries	Diffuse cerebral swelling: MVAs, falls Subdural hematoma: abuse, falls Skull fractures: MVAs, falls, abuse, sledding
Long bones	Salter-Harris fractures (prior to puberty) Periosteum is stronger and allows bone to bend, leading to greenstick fractures	Long bone fractures: falls, MVAs, abuse, sports

MVA, motor vehicle accident.

Mechanisms of Injury: Infant (birth to 1 year old)

Common Mechanisms of Injury

- Airway compromise
  - Choking
  - Strangulation
  - Suffocation
  - Foreign body ingestion
- Child abuse
  - Shaken baby syndrome
- Falls
- Burns (scalds or flame)
- Drownings
- Poisonings
- Baby walkers
- Motor vehicle–related injuries
- With or without the proper use/placement of car seats

INJURY PATTERN	RISK FACTORS	ASSOCIATED INJURIES
Abdomen	Pliable pelvic girdle does not protect internal organs Portion of bowel adheres to spine Organs easily crushed between bony structure and injury object	Laceration, fracture, rupture of solid organs (liver, spleen, kidney): MVAs, abuse, falls Hematoma, perforation of hollow organs (esophagus, stomach, intestines): MVAs, physical abuse
Chest	Tongue large in relation to oral cavity Narrow airway Obligate nose breather Short trachea Pliable rib cage Mobile mediastinal structures Absence of valves in superior and inferior venae cavae	Respiratory arrest: airway compromise, foreign body ingestion, obstruction Pneumothorax: MVAs, falls, abuse Pulmonary/cardiac contusion: MVAs, falls

(continued)

INJURY PATTERN	RISK FACTORS	ASSOCIATED INJURIES
Head	Head large in proportion to body Poor head control as a result of weak neck muscles Pliable body structures and vessels predispose infant to diffuse head injury	Skull fractures: abuse, falls Subdural hematoma: abuse Retinal hemorrhages: abuse, traumatic asphyxia Diffuse cerebral swelling: MVAs, abuse, falls High cervical fracture: MVAs

MVA, motor vehicle accident.

APPENDIX Q

Drugs of Abuse

DRUG NAME/ TYPE	STREET NAME	METHOD USED	PHYSICAL EFFECTS	MENTAL EFFECTS
Alcohol (a CNS depressant)	Booze, hooch, juice, brew	Swallowed in liquid form	Blurred vision; slurred speech, altered coordination; heart, liver, and brain damage; addiction; ulcers (gastric and esophageal); blackouts; anemia; hypoglycemia; Wernicke-Korsakoff syndrome; oral cancer; fetal alcohol syndrome; death	Scrambles thought process, impairs judgment, causes memory loss, alters perception, causes delirium, apathy
Cocaine (a CNS stimulant)	Coke, c-dust, snow, toot, white lady, blow, rock(s), crack, flake, big "C," happy dust, Bernice, fluff, caine, coconut, icing, mojo, zip, snow white, powder, Yeyo, Charlie, nose candy, happy trails	Smoked/free based; inhaled/ snorted; injected; swallowed in powder, pill, or rock form	Rapidly metabolized, producing a brief high of <30 minutes; chronic use results in cocaine psychosis, intense psychological dependence; dilated pupils; profuse sweating; runny nose; dry mouth; tachycardia; hypertension; insomnia; anorexia; damage to nasal septum, heart, and lungs; death from overdose	Euphoria, illusion of mental or physical power, extreme mood swings, restlessness, hallucinations, paranoia, psychosis, severe depression, anxiety, formication

(continued)

DRUG NAME/TYPE	STREET NAME	METHOD USED	PHYSICAL EFFECTS	MENTAL EFFECTS
CNS depressants—Barbiturates: mephobarbital, phenobarbital, amobarbital, secobarbital, pentobarbital, sodium pentothal	Reds, barbs, yellow jackets, red devils, blue devils, yellow submarine, blues and reds, idiot pills, sleepers, stumblers, downers	Intravenous injection, suppository, swallowed in pill form	Drowsiness, slurred speech, skeletal muscle relaxation, poor muscle control, nausea, slowed reaction time, involuntary eye movements, hypotension, bradycardia, bradypnea, constricted pupils, clammy skin, loss of appetite, crosses the placental wall (addiction is passed to the baby); withdrawal is prolonged and severe: symptoms range from temporary psychosis to cardiac arrest; cellulitis at injection site; chronic use results in extreme psychological and physical addiction; death from overdose	Confusion, impaired judgment, impaired performance, anxiety, and tension followed by a sense of calm, mood swings, forgetfulness
CNS depressants—Nonbarbiturates: methaqualone (Quaalude)	Downers, ludes, soapers, wallbangers, lemmons, 300s, lovers, quack, 714s, bandits, Beiruts, qua, blou bulle, ewings, quad flamingos, flowers, genuines, mandies	Swallowed in pill form	Same as barbiturates; physically and psychologically addictive; withdrawal is *very* difficult; severe interaction with alcohol; death from overdose	Same as barbiturates

(continued)

DRUG NAME/TYPE	STREET NAME	METHOD USED	PHYSICAL EFFECTS	MENTAL EFFECTS
CNS depressants—Benzodiazepines (reduce tension and anxiety without sedating): diazepam, chlordiazepoxide, lorazepam, oxazepam, alprazolam	Downers	Injection, swallowed in pill form	Decreased reflex action, vision changes, muscle relaxation, hypotension, bradycardia, slurred speech, drowsiness, blurred vision; prolonged use causes severe physical and psychological addiction	Alteration in spatial judgment and sense of time, sense of calm, impaired judgment, confusion, depression, hallucinations
CNS depressants—Non-benzodiazepine sedative hypnotics: zolpidem, eszopiclone, zaleplon	R zombie pills, xannies, Z-bars, bricks, zanbars, xanbars	Swallowed	Blurry vision, constipation, diarrhea, dizziness, drowsiness, headache, joint pain, lack of balance, nausea/vomiting, neuropathy, tinnitus, sleepwalking, sleep driving, bradycardia, bradypnea, loss of consciousness, coma	Hallucinations

(continued)

HALLUCINOGENS: DRUGS THAT ALTER PERCEPTIONS OF REALITY

DRUG NAME/TYPE	STREET NAME	METHOD USED	PHYSICAL EFFECTS	MENTAL EFFECTS
PCP (phencyclidine)	Angel dust, killer, black whack, supergrass, peace pill, sherms, superweed, DOA, CJ, goon dust, dust joint, live one, mad dog, T-buzz, wobble weed, zombie	Swallowed in pill form Sprayed on a cigarette and smoked	Drooling, nystagmus, restlessness, incoordination, rigid muscles, tachycardia, hypertension, superhuman strength, dulled sensations to touch and pain, impaired speech; death is common from accidents, not from overdose; a "trip" is a cycle of stimulation, depression, hallucination, and then repeats itself, lasting 2–14 hours	Disorientation, amnesia, anxiety, depression, confusion, agitation, violent behavior, hostility, suicidal urges, extreme personality changes
LSD (lysergic acid diethylamide)	Acid, blue heaven, instant zen, purple hearts, pure love, sugar cubes, tail lights	Swallowed in liquid form, dropped on sugar cube, sprayed on paper tablet	Nausea, tachycardia, tachypnea, hyperthermia, hypertension, dilated pupils, diaphoresis, palpitations, incoordination; trips last 4–14 hours; heightens all five senses	Altered perception of reality, psychotic disturbances, paranoia, synesthesia, hallucinations, mood swings, terrifying flashbacks
Mescaline, psilocybin mushrooms	Mesc, moon, peyote, buttons	Swallowed in natural form	Same as LSD	Same as LSD

(continued)

HALLUCINOGENS: DRUGS THAT ALTER PERCEPTIONS OF REALITY (cont.)

DRUG NAME/TYPE	STREET NAME	METHOD USED	PHYSICAL EFFECTS	MENTAL EFFECTS
Inhalants: volatile solvents (gasoline, airplane glue, paint thinner, dry cleaner fluid, degreasers, correction fluids, felt-tip markers)	Air blast, bagging, bang, bullet bolt, highball, huffing, glading, aimies, bolt, dusting, snot balls	Inhaled or sniffed using a paper bag, plastic bag, or rag	Incoordination, impaired vision, neuropathy, muscle weakness, anemia, vertigo, headache, weight loss, nausea, vomiting, sneezing, coughing, nosebleeds, slurred speech, tachycardia, fatigue, dilated pupils, chemical smell on breath; brain, liver, and bone marrow damage; death by anoxia	Memory and thought impairment, depression, aggression, hostility, paranoia, abusive behavior, mood swings, withdrawal from family and friends, violent behavior
Gases: nitrous oxide, chloroform, halothane	Laughing gas, whippets, buzz bomb, nitro	Inhaled or sniffed by mask or balloons	Headache, nausea/vomiting, shivering, fatigue, excessive sweating	Euphoria, relaxation, calmness, episodes of laughter
Nitrites: amyl nitrite, butyl nitrite, cyclohexyl nitrate	Poppers, snappers, pearls, aimies, bolt, climax, thrust	Inhaled or sniffed from gauze or ampules	Instead of acting on the CNS system, nitrites dilate blood vessels, relax muscles, act as sexual enhancers, damage to liver, heart, kidneys, brain, and bone marrow; dizziness	Hallucinations
Marijuana/hashish (a CNS depressant)	Joint, grass, hash, pot, "J," Maryjane, reefer, Colombian locoweed, love weed	Smoked, eaten	Interference with psychological maturation, psychological dependence	Sensory distortion, decrease in motivation, forgetfulness, confusion, anxiety, paranoia

(continued)

NARCOTICS: NATURAL OR SYNTHETIC DRUGS THAT CONTAIN OR RESEMBLE OPIUM; CNS DEPRESSANTS

DRUG NAME/TYPE	STREET NAME	METHOD USED	PHYSICAL EFFECTS	MENTAL EFFECTS
Dilaudid	Dillys, cowboys	Swallowed as pills or in liquid form, injected	Drowsiness, lethargy, hypotension, bradycardia	Forgetfulness, sedation, sense of peace
Percodan	Perks, pink spoons	Swallowed as pills	Adrenal insufficiency, nausea, vomiting, anorexia, fatigue, weakness, dizziness, low blood pressure, muscle weakness	Depression, hallucinations, confusion
Demerol	Demmies	Swallowed in pill or liquid form, snorted, injected	Hypotension, bradycardia, bradypnea, drowsiness, nausea, constipation, hypothermia, constricted pupils, slurred speech	Confusion, mood changes
Methadone	Dollies, dolls, amidone, fizzies, meth, phy, junk, metho, jungle juice	Swallowed in pill form, snorting, smoking, injection	Fatigue, dizziness, blurred vision, respiratory depression, seizures, hypotension	Confusion, agitation, hallucinations
Codeine	Schoolboy, cody, threes, fours	Swallowed in pill or liquid form	Liver damage, insomnia, seizures, coma, respiratory depression, nausea/vomiting	Irritability, emotional instability, extreme fatigue

(continued)

247 | Appendix Q

NARCOTICS: NATURAL OR SYNTHETIC DRUGS THAT CONTAIN OR RESEMBLE OPIUM; CNS DEPRESSANTS (cont.)

DRUG NAME/TYPE	STREET NAME	METHOD USED	PHYSICAL EFFECTS	MENTAL EFFECTS
Morphine	Mojo, morphy, mud, dreamer, Miss Emma	Smoked, intravenous injection, swallowed	Drowsiness, headache, dry mouth, abdominal cramps, seizures, nausea/vomiting, constricted pupils	Nervousness, euphoria, calmness, confusion, memory loss, stupor, irritability, agitation, hallucinations
Heroin	Horse, junk, dope, blanco, black pearl, bonita, smack		Warm sensation, dry mouth, nausea/vomiting, diarrhea, itching, drowsiness, bradycardia, bradypnea, coma, brain damage	Euphoria, mental blunting, emotional instability, insomnia
Fentanyl A potent synthetic opioid analgesic, 80–500 times stronger than morphine Becomes deadly when mixed with other drugs such as heroin or cocaine	Apache, fenty, he-man, white girl, birria (when mixed with heroin), China white, King Ivory	Patches, oral or nasal spray, lozenges, injection	Bowel obstruction, tremors, seizures, bradypnea, weakened immune system, coma, cardiac arrest	Delusions, hallucinations, personality changes, paranoia, confusion, social withdrawal, irritability

(continued)

CNS STIMULANTS

DRUG NAME/TYPE	STREET NAME	METHOD USED	PHYSICAL EFFECTS	MENTAL EFFECTS
Amphetamines: Benzedrine, Biphetamine Dextroamphetamines: Dexedrine, Synatan, Appetral Methamphetamines: Methedrine, Desoxyn, Ambar	Hi speed, lip poppers, speckled birds Dexies, brownies, brown and clears Speed, meth, crystal, crank, crypto, ice, yellow bam	Pill form, injected, snorted	Anorexia, tachycardia, palpitations, hypertension, inability to sleep, nasal and bronchial passages enlarge, restricted cerebral blood flow, dilated pupils, sweating, restlessness, muscle tremors, rapid and garbled speech, excessive activity, brain/liver/kidney/lung damage, seizures, stroke, coma, death	Extreme exhilaration, inflated confidence, irritability, volatile and aggressive behavior, nervousness, mood swings, hallucinations, paranoia, formication, psychosis, hypomania
Herbal stimulants (ephedra)	Ultimate Xphoria, herbal ecstasy, legal weed, buzz tablets, cloud 9, black lemonade, brainalizer, fungalore, herbal XTC, planet X, brain wash, buzz tablets, fukola cola, love potion #69	Pill, powder, liquid	Same as above; often marketed as safe and legal alternatives to street drugs; increased sexual sensation, higher energy level, tachycardia, sweating, body tremors, dilated pupils, muscle spasms, grinding of teeth, hypertension	Extreme exhilaration and stimulation, inflated confidence, reduced inhibitions, euphoria, irritability, volatile and aggressive behavior, nervousness, mood swings, hallucinations, paranoia, formication, psychosis, hypomania

(continued)

CNS STIMULANTS (cont.)

DRUG NAME/TYPE	STREET NAME	METHOD USED	PHYSICAL EFFECTS	MENTAL EFFECTS
Anesthetics Gamma hydroxybutyrate (GHB): also known as the "date rape drug"	Liquid X, liquid ecstasy, water, "G," easy lay	Oral	Slurred speech, ataxia, nausea/vomiting, bradycardia or tachycardia, hypotension, hypothermia; cardiac arrest, respiratory arrest, seizures, incontinences of stool and urine, coma	Memory loss, mood swings, amnesia, sleepiness, stupor, hallucinations, confusion, agitation
Ketamine (tranquilizer and hallucinogenic)	K, super K, special K, God, jet, honey oil, blast, gas	Injected, snorted, smoked, oral, rectal	Sweating, slurred speech, muscle rigidity, blank stare, tachycardia, loss of muscle coordination, hypertension, excess strength, seizures	Euphoria, paranoia, anxiety, disorientation, violence, agitation, insomnia, delusions, pain relief, intoxication, hallucinations, confusion, psychosis, symptoms similar to schizophrenia

CNS, central nervous system.

Poisonings

American Association of Poison Control Centers: (800) 222-1222

SUBSTANCE AND COMMON/STREET NAME	CLINICAL SIGNS AND SYMPTOMS
Acetaminophen Tylenol	Nausea, vomiting, anorexia, malaise, oliguria, increased liver enzymes Diffuse abdominal pain that localizes to the right upper quadrant
Alcohol	Sedation, relaxation, euphoria, memory loss, poor judgment, ataxia, slurred speech, nausea, vomiting, obtundation, coma In children, hypoglycemia also occurs
Amphetamines **Prescription:** Ritalin, Adderall, Dexedrine, Concerta, Vyvanse, Strattera, Focalin **Illegal:** ice, crank, ecstasy, crystal meth, MDMA, speed, speedball (when mixed with heroin)	CNS: agitation, delirium, hyperactivity, tremors, dizziness, mydriasis, CVA, headache, hyperreflexia, brain damage, seizures, coma, death Psychiatric: euphoria, paranoia, aggressive behavior, anxiety, hallucinations, compulsive repetitious actions, psychosis Cardiopulmonary: palpitations, hypertensive crisis, tachycardia, reflex bradycardia, dysrhythmias, myocardial infarction, aortic dissection, pulmonary edema, respiratory distress
Anticholinergics Antihistamines, antiparkinsonian, tricyclic antidepressants, antipsychotics, antispasmodics	Classic toxidrome: • "mad as a hatter" (hallucinations, confusion, confusion) • "hot as a hare" (hyperthermia) • "red as a beet" (flushed skin, tachycardia) • "dry as a bone" (dry skin and mucous membranes) • "blind as a bat" (blurry vision)
Arsenic	Acute ingestion: severe hemorrhagic gastroenteritis, bone marrow suppression, encephalopathy, cardiomyopathy, pulmonary edema, cardiac dysrhythmia Chronic exposure: weakness, anorexia, hyperkeratosis, hyperpigmentation, hepatic injury, respiratory irritation, perforated nasal septum, tremor, peripheral neuropathy, cancer, diabetes, heart disease, neurotoxicity, birth defects, developmental delays in children

(continued)

SUBSTANCE AND COMMON/STREET NAME	CLINICAL SIGNS AND SYMPTOMS
Barbiturates **Prescription:** Pentothal, Nembutal, Seconal, Mysoline, phenobarbital **Illegal:** downers, nembies, purple hearts, reds, rainbows	CNS: lethargy, slurred speech, incoordination, ataxia, coma, hyporeflexia, nystagmus, stupor Cardiopulmonary: hypotension, bradycardia, respiratory depression, apnea Other: rhabdomyolysis, compartment syndrome, hypoglycemia
Benzodiazepines Xanax, Librium, Clonopin, Valium, Ativan, Versed	CNS: nystagmus, miosis, diplopia, slurred speech, amnesia, ataxia, confusion, somnolence, depressed deep tendon reflexes, dyskinesia, paradoxical agitation Cardiopulmonary: hypotension, bradycardia, paradoxical tachycardia, respiratory depression, aspiration Other: hypothermia, rhabdomyolysis, skin necrosis
Beta-blockers Atenolol (Tenormin), metoprolol (Lopressor), propranolol	CNS: seizures, coma, CNS depression, disorientation Cardiopulmonary: hypotension, bradycardia, cardiac conduction delays, heart block, heart failure, bronchospasm, pulmonary edema, respiratory depression Other: hypoglycemia
Calcium-channel blockers Cardizem, Procardia, Calan SR	CNS: syncope, CNS depression, rare seizure, coma Cardiopulmonary: severe bradycardia, atrioventricular block, intraventricular conduction delays, ventricular dysrhythmias, congestive heart failure, respiratory depression, pulmonary edema Other: hyperglycemia, nausea, vomiting, ileus, hypotension, metabolic acidosis
Carbamazepine Oral antiseizure medications with a structure similar to that of tricyclic antidepressants	CNS: ataxia, dizziness, drowsiness, nystagmus, hallucinations, combativeness, coma, seizures Cardiopulmonary: respiratory depression, aspiration pneumonia, hypotension, conduction disturbances, supraventricular tachycardia, bradycardia, EKG changes Other: urinary retention, hyponatremia, myoclonus
Carbon monoxide	CNS: headache, dizziness, ataxia, confusion, acute encephalopathy, syncope, seizures, coma Cardiopulmonary: chest pain, palpitations, dyspnea, myocardial infarction, tachycardia, hypotension Other: nausea, vomiting, blurred vision, retinal hemorrhage, lactic acidosis, rhabdomyolysis, death

(continued)

SUBSTANCE AND COMMON/STREET NAME	CLINICAL SIGNS AND SYMPTOMS
Chloral hydrate **Prescription:** Noctec, Felsules **Illegal:** Mickey Finn, knockout drops	CNS: headache, lightheadedness, ataxia, hyporeflexia, confusion, seizures, sedation Cardiopulmonary: hypotension, ventricular and supraventricular dysrhythmias, bradypnea Other: nausea, vomiting, abdominal pain, rash, pear-like breath odor
Cyanide Can occur with smoke inhalation from fires, chronic ingestion of some foods, or as a chemical warfare agent	CNS: headache, confusion, syncope, seizures, coma, agitation, CNS stimulation Cardiopulmonary: tachycardia/hypertension, bradycardia/hypotension, myocardial infarction, pulmonary embolus, ventricular dysrhythmia, dyspnea, cardiac arrest Other: nausea, vomiting, abdominal pain, odor of almonds
Digoxin	CNS: colored visual halos, blurred vision, agitation, lethargy, seizures, psychosis, hallucinations Cardiopulmonary: hypotension, cardiovascular collapse, bradycardia, AV block, SA block, paroxysmal atrial tachycardia, congestive heart failure Other: nausea, vomiting, diarrhea, abdominal pain, thrombocytopenia
Ethylene glycol Antifreeze	CNS: ataxia, slurred speech, irritability, cerebral edema, brain damage, convulsions, coma Cardiopulmonary: tachycardia, bradycardia, hypotension, hypertension, pulmonary edema Other: nausea, vomiting, abdominal pain, hematemesis, acute renal failure, myalgia, hypocalcemia
Hallucinogens Lysergic acid diethylamide Dimethyltryptamine Tetrahydrocannabinol MDMA Peyote cactus	CNS: restlessness, anxiety, incipient dread, distortions of reality, helplessness, coma, hyperreflexia Cardiopulmonary: tachycardia, hypertension, dysrhythmias, tachypnea, respiratory arrest Other: nausea, vomiting, hyperpyrexia, coagulopathies
Hydrocarbons Gasoline, kerosene, paint thinner, lamp oil, etc. Recreational inhalation of these as well as glue, spray paint, refrigerants	CNS: intoxication, headache, euphoria, slurred speech, lethargy, coma Cardiopulmonary: respiratory distress, cyanosis, aspiration pneumonitis, tachycardia, dysrhythmia Other: mucosal irritation, gastritis, diarrhea, acute renal failure, hepatic toxicity

(continued)

SUBSTANCE AND COMMON/STREET NAME	CLINICAL SIGNS AND SYMPTOMS
Hypoglycemic agents • Sulfonylureas (glipizide, glyburide, gliclazide, glimepiride) • Meglitinides (repaglinide and nateglinide) • Biguanides (metformin) • Thiazolidinediones (rosiglitazone, pioglitazone) • Alpha-glucosidase inhibitors (acarbose, miglitol, voglibose) • DPP-4 inhibitors (sitagliptin, saxagliptin, vildagliptin, linagliptin, alogliptin) • SGLT2 inhibitors (dapagliflozin and canagliflozin) • Cycloset (bromocriptine)	CNS: headache, blurred vision, anxiety, irritability, confusion, stupor, coma, seizures Cardiopulmonary: respiratory distress, apnea, palpitations, tachycardia, hypertension, premature ventricular contractions Other: nausea, facial flushing, hypoglycemia, facial flushing, pallor
Iron	CNS: lethargy, seizures, coma Cardiopulmonary: tachycardia, tachypnea, hypotension Other: vomiting, abdominal pain, gastrointestinal bleeding, diarrhea, renal failure, hepatic necrosis
Isoniazid	CNS: ataxia, hyperreflexia, agitation, hallucinations, psychosis, coma, seizures Cardiopulmonary: hypotension, tachycardia, shock, respiratory depression, Kussmaul respirations Other: hyperthermia, nausea, vomiting, severe anion gap, rhabdomyolysis, hepatic toxicity
Lead (adult)	CNS: headache, confusion, altered mental status, seizures, nerve entrapment, motor neuropathy Cardiopulmonary/reproductive: hypertension, alterations in sperm count and quality Other: anorexia, dyspepsia, constipation, renal failure
Lead (pediatric)	CNS: cognitive dysfunction, decreased IQ, encephalopathy, irritability, headache, coma Hematologic: anemia, basophilic stippling Other: nausea, vomiting, abdominal pain, mild hearing loss
Lithium	CNS: lethargy, confusion, tremor, ataxia, slurred speech, hyperreflexia, clonus, dystonia Cardiopulmonary: EKG changes, respiratory failure Other: nausea, vomiting, diarrhea, diabetes insipidus, leukocytosis

(continued)

SUBSTANCE AND COMMON/STREET NAME	CLINICAL SIGNS AND SYMPTOMS
Methanol Windshield washer fluid	CNS: inebriation, ataxia, seizures, coma, blurred vision, dilated pupils, headache, confusion Cardiopulmonary: hyperpnea, hypotension Other: metabolic acidosis, nausea, vomiting, abdominal pain, renal failure
Nonsteroidal anti-inflammatory agents (aspirin, ibuprofen, indomethacin)	CNS: drowsiness, dizziness, lethargy, seizures Cardiopulmonary: hypotension, tachycardia, hyperventilation, apnea Other: nausea, vomiting, abdominal pain, acute renal failure, metabolic acidosis
Organophosphates Insecticides	CNS: headache, dizziness, tremors, anxiety, weakness, agitation, incoordination, convulsions, coma Cardiopulmonary: hypotension, bradycardia, atrioventricular block, asystole, bronchospasm, pulmonary edema, respiratory failure Other: miosis, anorexia, abdominal cramps, salivation, lacrimation, blurry vision
Phencyclidines (PCP, Angel Dust, Crystal)	CNS: impaired judgment, agitation, violent behavior, psychosis, paranoia, coma, seizures, dyskinesia Cardiopulmonary: hypertension, tachycardia, apnea Other: hyperthermia, acute renal failure, hypoglycemia
Phenothiazines Chlorpromazine Clozapine Fluphenazine Haloperidol Loxapine Molindone Perphenazine Pimozide Prochlorperazine Thioridazine Thiothixene Trifluoperazine Promethazine	CNS: agitation, seizures, coma, extrapyramidal signs, tardive dyskinesia, confusion Cardiopulmonary: respiratory depression, pulmonary edema, tachycardia, EKG changes, ventricular tachycardia, hypertension, hypotension Other: hyperthermia, priapism, acute renal failure, constipation, ileus, agranulocytosis, anemia
Phenytoin	CNS: ataxia, nystagmus, cortical depression, confusion, slurred speech, coma, seizures Cardiopulmonary: hypotension, bradycardia, myocardial depression with rapid intravenous infusion Other: nausea, vomiting

(continued)

SUBSTANCE AND COMMON/STREET NAME	CLINICAL SIGNS AND SYMPTOMS
Salicylates	CNS: tinnitus, deafness, delirium, seizures, coma, agitation, lethargy, confusion, cerebral edema Cardiopulmonary: hypotension, shock, tachypnea, noncardiac pulmonary edema, hyperventilation Other: nausea, vomiting, hepatic injury, acute renal insufficiency, hematemesis
Sympathomimetics Ephedrine Amphetamines Methamphetamine Ephedra alkaloids Methamphetamine Cocaine	CNS: anxiety, headache, agitation, altered mentation, diaphoresis, stroke, seizures Cardiopulmonary: palpitations, chest pain, myocardial ischemia, tachydysrhythmias, hypertension Other: dilated pupils, dry mucous membranes, urinary retention, hyperthermia
Theophylline	CNS: tremor, agitation, nervousness, seizures Cardiopulmonary: hypotension, tachycardia, tachypnea, hypertension, dysrhythmias Other: nausea, vomiting, abdominal pain, hypokalemia, hyperglycemia, leukocytosis
Toluene/toluol An aromatic hydrocarbon found in paints, chemicals, and glue	CNS: depression, euphoria, ataxia, seizures, insomnia, brain damage, headache, coma Cardiopulmonary: sudden cardiac death, dilated cardiomyopathy, myocardial infarction, chemical pneumonitis Other: renal failure, rhabdomyolysis, hematemesis, abdominal pain, electrolyte imbalance, liver damage, blurry vision, bloody emesis, and/or diarrhea
Tricyclic antidepressants Amitriptyline, nortriptyline, and doxepin	CNS: agitation, tremors, seizures, drowsiness, lethargy, coma, ataxia, mania, dilated pupils Cardiopulmonary: hypotension, tachycardia, bradycardia, EKG changes, dysrhythmias Other: urinary retention, priapism, leukopenia, nausea, vomiting, hyperthermia

AV, atrioventricular; CNS, central nervous system; CVA, cerebrovascular accident; MDMA, methylenedioxy-methamphetamine; SA, sinoatrial; SGLT2, sodium-glucose cotransporter-2.

APPENDIX S

Biological Agents/Chemical Agents

BIOLOGICAL AGENTS

Agent and Incu-bation Period	Signs, Symptoms, Sequelae, and Mode of Acquisition	Source	Vaccine Available	Contagious Be-tween Humans	Treatment	Comments
Anthrax (inhaled): *Bacillus anthracis;* 7 days post exposure	Resembles a common cold (fever, cough, malaise) that progresses to severe dyspnea, diaphoresis, stridor, cyanosis, and shock Chest radiograph shows a mediastinal widening Gram-positive bacilli seen on blood smear and culture Hemorrhagic mediastinitis, thoracic lymphadenitis, and/or meningitis Inhalation of spores from contaminated animal products	Infected animal tissue Spores can live in the soil for years Biological warfare agent	Yes; approved for ages 18–65 Three injections given 2 weeks apart, followed by three more injections at 6, 12, and 18 months	Extremely unlikely	Early treatment is essential Penicillin Doxycycline Ciprofloxacin Special considerations for treatment of children, elderly, and pregnant women	90%–100% of cases are fatal

(continued)

Agent and Incubation Period	Signs, Symptoms, Sequelae, and Mode of Acquisition	Source	Vaccine Available	Contagious Between Humans	Treatment	Comments
Anthrax (cutaneous): *B. anthracis*; 7 days post exposure	Spores enter the skin Infection more likely with a cut or abrasion on the skin Infections begin with a raised, itchy bump that resembles a bug bite Within 1–2 days, a vesicle develops, followed by a painless ulcer 1–3 cm in diameter with a black necrotic center Lymph glands in the adjacent area may swell	Infected animal tissue, hair, fur, hides, leather Spores can live in the soil for years Biological warfare agent	Yes; approved for ages 18–65 Three injections given 2 weeks apart, followed by three more injections at 6, 12, and 18 months	Rare, but can occur	Early treatment is essential Penicillin Doxycycline Ciprofloxacin Special consideration for treatment of children, elderly, and pregnant women	Death rare if treated 20% of untreated cases are fatal

(continued)

Agent and Incu-bation Period	Signs, Symptoms, Sequelae, and Mode of Acquisition	Source	Vaccine Available	Contagious Be-tween Humans	Treatment	Comments
Anthrax (intestinal): *B. anthracis;* 7 days post exposure	Early symptoms: nausea, vomiting, malaise, anorexia, fever, acute in-flammation of the GI tract Advanced symptoms: ab-dominal pain, vomiting blood, severe diarrhea Illness progresses rapidly Eating undercooked contami-nated food	Infected animal tissue Spores can live in the soil for years Biological war-fare agent	Yes; approved for ages 18–65 Three injections given 2 weeks apart, followed by three more injections at 6, 12, and 18 months	Extremely unlikely	Early treatment is essential Penicillin Doxycycline Ciprofloxacin Special consid-erations for treatment of children, elderly, and pregnant women Antitoxin avail-able from CDC; must be adminis-tered early in course of disease Supportive care	25%–75% of cases are fatal

(continued)

Agent and Incubation Period	Signs, Symptoms, Sequelae, and Mode of Acquisition	Source	Vaccine Available	Contagious Between Humans	Treatment	Comments
Botulism (food-borne): *Clostridium botulinum*; incubation depends on amount of toxin and rate of toxin absorption: ranges from 2 hours to 8 days	Early symptoms: abdominal cramps, nausea, vomiting, diarrhea, and difficulty seeing, speaking, swallowing Double or blurred vision, drooping eyelids, slurred speech, dry mouth Progresses to an acute, afebrile, symmetric, descending flaccid paralysis with multiple cranial nerve palsies, coma The most poisonous substance known; a major bioweapon threat due to its extreme potency, lethality, and ease of production, transport, and misuse	Contaminated food from restaurants or home-canned sources Bacteria commonly found in the soil	Botulinum toxoid is available, but supplies are scarce and mass outbreaks of disease are rare	No		Presents public health emergency Mortality rate = 8%

(continued)

Agent and Incubation Period	Signs, Symptoms, Sequelae, and Mode of Acquisition	Source	Vaccine Available	Contagious Between Humans	Treatment	Comments
Botulism (inhaled): *C. botulinum;* incubation depends on amount of toxin and rate of toxin absorption, ranges from 12 to 80 hours	Ptosis, diplopia, blurred vision, dysarthria, dysphonia, dysphagia Progresses to an acute, afebrile, symmetric, descending flaccid paralysis with multiple cranial nerve palsies, coma The most poisonous substance known; a major bioweapon threat due to its extreme potency, lethality, and ease of production, transport, and misuse	An aerosolized form of the bacteria developed for use in bioterrorism	Botulinum toxoid is available, but supplies are scarce and mass outbreaks of disease are rare	No	Supportive care	Same as for food-borne botulism
Botulism (wound): *C. botulinum;* incubation depends on amount of toxin and rate of toxin absorption	Double or blurred vision, drooping eyelids, slurred speech, dry mouth Progresses to an acute, afebrile, symmetric, descending flaccid paralysis with multiple cranial nerve palsies, coma Will *not* penetrate intact skin	Bacteria found in soil In recent years, black tar heroin from California is a prime source	As for food-borne and inhaled botulism	No	Antitoxin available from CDC; must be administered early in course of disease Supportive care	Infectious disease that would *not* result from bioterrorism

(continued)

Agent and Incubation Period	Signs, Symptoms, Sequelae, and Mode of Acquisition	Source	Vaccine Available	Contagious Between Humans	Treatment	Comments
Botulism (intestinal): *C. botulinum*	Lethargy, poor feeding, constipation, weakness, crying, and poor muscle tone Occasionally, susceptible patients may harbor *C. botulinum* in their intestinal tract (most often occurs in infants)	Bacteria commonly found in the soil	As for food-borne and inhaled botulism	No	Supportive care Antitoxin is not routinely given for infant botulism	Infectious disease that would *not* result from bioterrorism
Brucellosis (food-borne): *Brucella* species; incubation is variable	Flu-like symptoms, such as fever, sweats, headache, back pain, weakness In severe cases, the patient may develop hepatitis, arthritis, spondylitis, anemia, leukopenia, thrombocytopenia, meningitis, uveitis, optic neuritis, papilledema, and endocarditis Chronic symptoms may include recurrent fevers, joint pain, and fatigue	Ingestion of contaminated milk, dairy, or animal products High risk in unpasteurized milk, cheese, and ice cream	None available for humans	Extremely rare, although may possibly be transmitted through breast milk, sexual contact, or tissue transplantation	Doxycycline and rifampin used in combination for 6 weeks Recovery takes a few weeks to several months	Mortality <2%

(continued)

Agent and Incubation Period	Signs, Symptoms, Sequelae, and Mode of Acquisition	Source	Vaccine Available	Contagious Between Humans	Treatment	Comments
Brucellosis (inhaled): *Brucella* species	Same as for food-borne brucellosis	Inhalation of aerosolized *Brucella*	None available for humans	Same as for food-borne brucellosis	Same as for food-borne brucellosis	Same as for food-borne brucellosis
Brucellosis (wound): *Brucella* species	Same as for food-borne brucellosis	Transmitted via skin abrasions while handling infected animals	None available for humans	Same as for food-borne brucellosis	Same as for food-borne brucellosis	Same as for food-borne brucellosis
Pneumonic plague: *Yersinia pestis*; incubation is 1–6 days post exposure	Early signs are fever, headache, weakness, dyspnea, and productive cough (bloody or watery sputum)	Bacteria carried by rodents and their fleas	None at this time; however, research is underway	Occurs through respiratory droplets during face-to-face contact	Early treatment is important Streptomycin Tetracycline Doxycycline	Death can occur in as little as 2–4 days

(continued)

Agent and Incubation Period	Signs, Symptoms, Sequelae, and Mode of Acquisition	Source	Vaccine Available	Contagious Between Humans	Treatment	Comments
Pneumonic plague (*cont.*)	May see nausea, vomiting, abdominal pain, or diarrhea Acutely swollen and painful lymph nodes appear on the second day of infection, and the overlying skin is erythematous Pneumonia progresses over 2–4 days followed by septic shock and death	Bioweapon usage would occur after aerosolization of the bacteria			Special considerations for treatment of children, elderly, and pregnant women Respiratory precautions, prophylactic antibiotics for close contacts of patient	

(continued)

Agent and Incubation Period	Signs, Symptoms, Sequelae, and Mode of Acquisition	Source	Vaccine Available	Contagious Between Humans	Treatment	Comments
Smallpox: *Variola* virus; incubation is 7–17 days post exposure	Initial symptoms are high fever, fatigue, headaches, and back aches 2–3 days later, a rash appears in the mouth and on the face, arms, and legs, beginning as flat red lesions that evolve at the same rate; after a day or two, the lesions become pus-filled and begin to crust early in the second week; scabs fall off after 3–4 weeks Patients with smallpox are most infectious during the first week of illness, although they are contagious until all skin scabs are healed In people exposed to smallpox, the vaccine can be given within 4 days to lessen or prevent the illness	Infected saliva droplets	The United States has an emergency supply available	Occurs through respiratory droplets during face-to-face contact Can also be transmitted by contaminated clothing or bedding	No proven treatment, although research for antivirals continues. Supportive care includes IV fluids, antipyretics, antibiotics for secondary infections Patients should be placed in negative-pressure rooms; staff should use precautions to protect against spread of the disease	Mortality rate = 30%

(continued)

Agent and Incubation Period	Signs, Symptoms, Sequelae, and Mode of Acquisition	Source	Vaccine Available	Contagious Between Humans	Treatment	Comments
Tularemia: *Francisella tularensis*; incubation is 1–14 days post exposure	Initial symptoms are fever, pharyngitis, headache, body aches, and upper respiratory illness, rapidly progressing to bronchitis, pneumonia, pneumonitis, bacteremia; may see nausea, weight loss, malaise with continued illness Inhalation would have the greatest adverse public health consequences; release in a densely populated area would result in an abrupt onset of a sick population (but slower progression than anthrax or plague) A dangerous bioweapon due to its extreme infectivity, ease of dissemination, and substantial capacity to cause illness and death	Contaminated arthropods, soil, animals, water, and vegetation Humans become infected by direct contact, ingestion, or inhaled infective aerosols	Vaccine available; not fully approved for general use	No	Individual treatment drugs of choice: streptomycin, gentamicin Mass casualty treatment drugs of choice: doxycycline, ciprofloxacin Special considerations for children, pregnant women, and those with immunosuppression	Mortality rate is <2%

(continued)

Agent and Incu-bation Period	Signs, Symptoms, Sequelae, and Mode of Acquisition	Source	Vaccine Available	Contagious Be-tween Humans	Treatment	Comments
Viral hemor-rhagic fevers (VHF)	A severe multisystem syndrome in which the overall vascular system is damaged Initially, fever, fatigue, dizziness, muscle aches, weakness are seen Severe infections will pro-duce petechiae, internal bleeding, or bleeding from body orifices; syndrome progresses to shock, nervous system malfunction, coma, de-lirium, seizures, and/or renal failure A group of illnesses caused by several families of viruses: arenaviruses (Argentine, Bolivian, Lassa); bunyaviruses (Rift Valley, hantaviruses); filo-viruses (Ebola, Marburg); flaviviruses (tickborne, Kyasanur Forest)	Most VHFs are insect or ani-mal borne The vectors for Ebola and Marburg viruses are unknown Humans become infected through contact with rodent's bodily fluids or when bitten by an arthropod	Available only for yellow fever and Argentine hemorrhagic fever at this time No vaccines exist for the other VHFs	Humans may transmit some of these VHFs to other humans	There are no treatments for most of the VHFs Supportive care is given	Mortality rate varies with each VHF; most have a mortal-ity rate between 50% and 90%

(continued)

Agent and Incubation Period	Signs, Symptoms, Sequelae, and Mode of Acquisition	Source	Vaccine Available	Contagious Between Humans	Treatment	Comments
Q fever: *Coxiella burnetii*; incubation is 2–3 weeks post exposure	Sudden onset of high fevers (104°F–105°F), severe headache, malaise, myalgia, confusion, sore throat, chills, sweats, nonproductive cough, nausea, vomiting, diarrhea, abdominal pain, chest pain Fever lasts for 1–2 weeks 30%–50% of patients develop pneumonia This agent is highly infectious and resistant to heat, drying, and most disinfectants; it easily becomes airborne and is inhaled by humans and therefore is at risk of abuse by bioterrorists Chronic Q fever occurs when infection persists for >6 months; these patients are prone to endocarditis	Infected milk, urine, feces, amniotic fluid of animals Humans are infected by inhaling dried, contaminated particles Ingestion of contaminated milk may produce illness	A vaccine exists in Australia, although not commercially available in the United States	Rare	Q fever: doxycycline; most effective when started within first 3 days of illness Chronic Q fever: doxycycline with quinolones for at least 4 years or doxycycline with hydroxychloroquine for 1.5–3 years	Q fever: <2% mortality rate Chronic Q fever: 65% mortality rate

CDC, Centers for Disease Control and Prevention.

CHEMICAL AGENTS

Agents and Descriptions	Onset of Symptoms Post Exposure	Signs and Symptoms, Routes of Exposure	Action, Risks	Decontamination and Treatment
Nerve Agents				
Sarin: Pure liquid is clear, colorless, tasteless; becomes brown with aging	Immediately if inhaled; may be several hours if it touches the skin	Runny nose, watery eyes, drooling, blurred vision, headache, excessive sweating, chest tightness, difficulty breathing, nausea, vomiting, loss of bowel and bladder control, muscle cramps, twitching, confusion, convulsions, paralysis, and coma Can enter the body by inhalation, ingestion, through the eyes and skin	Chemicals that attack the nervous system by binding with acetylcholinesterase, allowing acetylcholine to overstimulate the glands and voluntary muscles until they fail Lethal; one drop on the skin can cause death in <15 minutes	**Skin:** Remove contaminated clothing (double-bag in plastic bags and seal) and wash skin with large amount of soap and water or 5% bleach. Rinse well with water. **Eyes:** Immediately flush eyes with water for 10–15 minutes; do *not* cover eyes with patches afterward. **Ingestion:** Do *not* induce vomiting. If patient alert and able to swallow, immediately administer activated charcoal.

(continued)

Agents and Descriptions	Onset of Symptoms Post Exposure	Signs and Symptoms, Routes of Exposure	Action, Risks	Decontamination and Treatment
Sarin (cont.)				**Vapor:** Remove outer clothing and place in sealed double-bag. Care for exposed skin as earlier. **Emergency treatment and antidotes:** Maintain airway, cardiac monitor, IVs, monitor vital signs. Follow ACLS protocols.
VX (thiophosphonate): Amber colored, tasteless, and odorless oily liquid	Onset of symptoms varies based on route of exposure VX absorbs very rapidly through the eyes At least 100 times more toxic than sarin when entering through the skin and twice as toxic by inhalation	Runny nose, watery eyes, drooling, excessive sweating, chest tightness, dyspnea, pinpoint pupils, nausea, vomiting, abdominal cramps, incontinence of bowel or bladder, twitching, headache, confusion, coma, or seizures	Kills by binding acetylcholinesterase; this causes constant stimulation of glands and voluntary muscles until ultimate fatigue and a cessation of breathing ability Extremely lethal and persistent; can last for months in cold weather; evaporates 1,500 times slower than water	**Skin:** Remove contaminated clothes and wash skin with large amounts of soap and water, 10% sodium carbonate, or 5% liquid household bleach. Rinse well with water. Administer antidote only if local sweating and muscular twitching are present.

(continued)

Agents and Descriptions	Onset of Symptoms Post Exposure	Signs and Symptoms, Routes of Exposure	Action, Risks	Decontamination and Treatment
VX (thiophosphonate) (*cont.*)		Can enter the body by inhalation, ingestion, through the eyes and skin Death can occur within 15 minutes of absorption of fatal dosage.		**Eyes:** *Immediately* flush eyes with water for 10–15 minutes, then place respiratory protective mask. Use antidote only if more symptoms than just miosis occur. VX is absorbed 100 times faster through the eyes than sarin. **Ingestion:** Do *not* induce vomiting. **Inhalation:** Use positive-pressure, full-face breathing mask. Do *not* perform mouth-to-mouth on a patient with VX exposure! Immediately administer nerve agent antidote. **Emergency treatment and antidotes:** Maintain airway, cardiac monitor, IVs, monitor vital signs. Follow ACLS protocols.

(*continued*)

Agents and Descriptions	Onset of Symptoms Post Exposure	Signs and Symptoms, Routes of Exposure	Action, Risks	Decontamination and Treatment
GF (cyclosarin): Colorless and odorless liquid in pure form	Depending on the dose, onset of symptoms within minutes or hours Rapid absorption through the eyes	Runny nose, miosis, headache, dyspnea, chest tightness, cough, drooling, excessive sweating, copious sinus secretions, nausea, vomiting, abdominal cramps, diarrhea, incontinence of bowel and bladder, muscle twitching and weakness, confusion, apnea, coma, death Can enter the body by inhalation, ingestion, through the eyes and skin	Organophosphorus compound, a lethal cholinesterase inhibitor similar in action to sarin	**Skin:** Remove contaminated clothes and wash skin with large amounts of soap and water, 10% sodium carbonate, or 5% liquid household bleach. Rinse well with water. Administer antidote only if local sweating and muscular twitching are present. **Eyes:** *Immediately flush eyes with water for 10–15 minutes, then place respiratory protective mask. Use antidote only if more symptoms than just miosis occur.* **Ingestion:** Do *not* induce vomiting. Immediately administer nerve agent antidote.

(continued)

Agents and Descriptions	Onset of Symptoms Post Exposure	Signs and Symptoms, Routes of Exposure	Action, Risks	Decontamination and Treatment
GF (cyclosarin) (*cont.*)				**Inhalation:** Use positive-pressure, full-face, self-contained breathing apparatus. For severe signs, immediately administer nerve agent antidote and oxygen. Do *not* perform mouth-to-mouth resuscitation if face is contaminated with GF. **Emergency treatment and antidotes:** Maintain airway, cardiac monitor, IVs, monitor vital signs. Follow ACLS protocols.

(*continued*)

Agents and Descriptions	Onset of Symptoms Post Exposure	Signs and Symptoms, Routes of Exposure	Action, Risks	Decontamination and Treatment
Pulmonary Agents				
Nitrogen oxide: Red/brown gas or a yellow liquid with pungent odor	The substance and vapor irritate the eyes, skin, and respiratory tract Effects may be delayed	Cough, wheezing, sore throat, dizziness, headache, sweating, vomiting, dyspnea, or redness at point of contact (eyes, skin) Can enter the body by inhalation or ingestion	Causes lung edema Exposure to high amounts can cause death	**Skin:** Rinse with plenty of water then remove contaminated clothing and rinse again. Refer for medical attention. **Eyes:** Flush eyes with water for 10–15 minutes (be sure to remove contact lenses), then refer for medical attention. **Ingestion:** Rinse mouth with copious amounts of water. **Inhalation:** Provide oxygen, place in sitting position. Seek medical evaluation.

(continued)

Agents and Descriptions	Onset of Symptoms Post Exposure	Signs and Symptoms, Routes of Exposure	Action, Risks	Decontamination and Treatment
Chlorine: Green/yellow gas with pungent odor	Effects may be delayed	Very corrosive effects Tearing of the eyes, cough, headache, sore throat, dyspnea, burning sensation, lung edema, frostbite, burns to the skin, nausea, eye pain, blurred vision Enters the body by inhalation	Corrosive effects to lungs, skin, and eyes Chronic exposure results in erosion of the teeth, chronic bronchitis Overexposure can cause death	**Skin:** Remove contaminated clothing, then rinse skin with plenty of water or a shower. Seek medical help for burns. **Eyes:** Flush eyes with water for 10–15 minutes (be sure to remove contact lenses), then refer for medical attention. **Inhalation:** Provide oxygen, place in sitting position. May need artificial ventilation. Seek medical evaluation.

(continued)

Agents and Descriptions	Onset of Symptoms Post Exposure	Signs and Symptoms, Routes of Exposure	Action, Risks	Decontamination and Treatment
Sulfur dioxide: Colorless gas or compressed liquefied gas with pungent odor	Inhalation symptoms may be delayed Contact with skin can cause immediate frostbite	Frostbite to the skin, eye pain with redness and severe burns, sore throat, cough, dyspnea, lung edema, reflex spasm of the larynx, respiratory arrest, death Enters the body by inhalation	Strong irritant to the eyes and respiratory tract Repeated or prolonged exposure can cause asthma	**Skin:** Remove contaminated clothing, then rinse with plenty of water. Do *not* remove clean clothing. Seek medical help for frostbite. **Eyes:** Flush eyes with water for 10–15 minutes (be sure to remove contact lenses), then refer for medical attention. **Inhalation:** Provide oxygen, place in sitting position. May need artificial ventilation. Seek medical evaluation.

(continued)

Agents and Descriptions	Onset of Symptoms Post Exposure	Signs and Symptoms, Routes of Exposure	Action, Risks	Decontamination and Treatment
Phosgene: Colorless gas, colorless to yellow compressed liquefied gas with characteristic odor	Inhalation symptoms may be delayed Contact with skin can cause immediate frostbite	Frostbite to the skin, eye pain with redness and severe burns, blurred vision, sore throat, cough, dyspnea, lung edema, death Enters the body by inhalation	Corrosive to skin, respiratory tract, and eyes Long-term exposure may result in lung fibrosis	**Skin:** Remove contaminated clothing, then rinse with plenty of water. Do *not* remove clean clothing. Seek medical help for frostbite. **Eyes:** Flush eyes with water for 10–15 minutes (be sure to remove contact lenses), then refer for medical attention. **Inhalation:** Provide oxygen, place in sitting position. May need artificial ventilation. Seek medical evaluation.

(continued)

Agents and Descriptions	Onset of Symptoms Post Exposure	Signs and Symptoms, Routes of Exposure	Action, Risks	Decontamination and Treatment
Titanium tetrachloride: Colorless to light yellow liquid with pungent odor	Symptoms may be delayed	Red painful eyes with burns, skin blisters, cough, dyspnea, chest tightness, abdominal pain, shock, coma Enters the body by inhalation or ingestion	Corrosive to skin, eyes, respiratory, and gastrointestinal tract; can cause permanent eye damage Long-term exposure may result in lung impairment	**Skin:** Remove contaminated clothing, rinse with plenty of water, then wash with soap and water **Eyes:** Flush eyes with water for 10–15 minutes (be sure to remove contact lenses), then refer for medical attention. **Ingestion:** Rinse mouth. Do *not* induce vomiting. Seek medical attention immediately **Inhalation:** Provide oxygen, place in sitting position. May need artificial ventilation. Seek medical evaluation.

(continued)

Agents and Descriptions	Onset of Symptoms Post Exposure	Signs and Symptoms, Routes of Exposure	Action, Risks	Decontamination and Treatment
Blister Agents				
Lewisite: Amber to dark brown liquid with a strong, penetrating geranium odor; the pure compound is a colorless, odorless, oily liquid	Immediate symptoms with eye exposure, inhalation, or ingestion Skin contact produces symptoms within 30 minutes	Eyelid swelling, severe eye pain, iritis, copious sinus drainage, violent sneezing, cough, frothing mucus, lung edema, large skin blisters and burns, diarrhea, hypothermia, hypotension Severe irritation and lung edema; can cause systemic poisoning, hemoconcentration, shock, and death Can enter the body by inhalation, ingestion, through the eyes and skin	Causes blindness within 1 minute of exposure Nonfatal hemolysis results in anemia Metabolites excreted by liver cause focal necrosis of liver, biliary passages, and intestine Long-term exposure can cause chronic lung impairment and cancer	**Skin:** Immediately wash skin and clothes with 5% sodium hypochlorite or household bleach within 1 minute of exposure, then cut and remove contaminated clothing. Rewash skin with 5% liquid household bleach. Then wash contaminated skin a third time with soap and water. **Eyes:** Immediately flush eyes with water for 10–15 minutes. **Ingestion:** Rinse mouth. Do *not* induce vomiting. Give patient milk to drink.

(continued)

Agents and Descriptions	Onset of Symptoms Post Exposure	Signs and Symptoms, Routes of Exposure	Action, Risks	Decontamination and Treatment
Lewisite (*cont.*)				**Inhalation:** Provide oxygen, place in sitting position. May need artificial ventilation. Do *not* perform mouth-to-mouth resuscitation if facial contamination has occurred.
Mustard gas: Pure liquid is colorless and odorless; agent-grade material is yellow, brown, or black with a sweet-type odor of garlic or horseradish	Rapid penetration of moist mucous membranes and skin Delayed severe symptoms of the respiratory tract	Severe tearing and pain of eyes with possible blindness, sneezing, coughing, anorexia, diarrhea, fever, skin blisters Can enter the body by inhalation, ingestion, or through the eyes and skin; tender skin, mucous membranes, and perspiration-covered skin are more vulnerable	Causes delayed severe damage to the respiratory tract and cytotoxic action on hematopoietic tissues Lethal doses are carcinogens and teratogens Distilled mustard is nearly pure, while mustard gas is only 70%–80% pure	**Skin:** Immediately wash skin and clothes with 5% sodium hypochlorite or household bleach within 1 minute of exposure, then cut and remove contaminated clothing. Flush skin again with 5% sodium hypochlorite solution, then wash contaminated skin a third time with soap and water.

(continued)

Agents and Descriptions	Onset of Symptoms Post Exposure	Signs and Symptoms, Routes of Exposure	Action, Risks	Decontamination and Treatment
Mustard gas (cont.)				**Eyes:** Immediately flush eyes with water for 10–15 minutes. Do not cover with bandages. Use dark goggles or glasses. **Ingestion:** Do *not* induce vomiting. Give patient milk to drink. **Inhalation:** Provide oxygen, place in sitting position. May need artificial ventilation. Do *not* perform mouth-to-mouth resuscitation if facial contamination has occurred.

(continued)

Agents and Descriptions	Onset of Symptoms Post Exposure	Signs and Symptoms, Routes of Exposure	Action, Risks	Decontamination and Treatment
Blood Agents				
Arsine: Colorless compressed liquefied gas with a characteristic odor	Immediate to delayed symptoms, depending on exposure	Causes immediate frostbite when contact made with eyes or skin Headache, confusion, dizziness, nausea, vomiting, abdominal pain, dyspnea, lung edema, kidney failure, damage to blood cells, death Enters the body by inhalation	Chronic exposure is carcinogenic to humans	**Skin:** Remove contaminated clothing, then rinse with plenty of water. Do *not* remove clean clothing. Seek medical help for frostbite. **Eyes:** Flush eyes with water for 10–15 minutes, follow with an immediate eye examination. **Inhalation:** Provide oxygen, place in sitting position. May need artificial ventilation.

(continued)

Agents and Descriptions	Onset of Symptoms Post Exposure	Signs and Symptoms, Routes of Exposure	Action, Risks	Decontamination and Treatment
Cyanogen chloride: Colorless compressed liquefied gas with a pungent odor	Effects of exposure may be delayed	Causes immediate frostbite when contact made with eyes or skin Sore throat, severe tearing, confusion, drowsiness, unconsciousness, nausea, vomiting, lung edema Enters the body by inhalation or absorbed through the skin	Overexposure results in death	**Skin:** Remove contaminated clothing, then rinse with plenty of water. Do *not* remove clean clothing. Seek medical help for frostbite. **Eyes:** Flush eyes with water for 10–15 minutes, follow with an immediate eye examination. **Inhalation:** Provide oxygen, place in sitting position. May need artificial ventilation.
Hydrogen chloride: Colorless compressed liquefied gas with a pungent odor	Highly corrosive; symptoms may begin immediately or be delayed	Corrosive, deep, severe burns to eyes and skin Sore throat, blurred vision, coughing, dyspnea, lung edema, burning sensation	Long-term exposure may cause erosion to the teeth or chronic bronchitis	**Skin:** Remove contaminated clothing, then rinse with plenty of water. Seek treatment for burns. **Eyes:** Flush eyes with water for 10–15 minutes; follow with an immediate eye examination.

(continued)

Agents and Descriptions	Onset of Symptoms Post Exposure	Signs and Symptoms, Routes of Exposure	Action, Risks	Decontamination and Treatment
Hydrogen chloride (*cont.*)		Enters the body through inhalation		**Inhalation:** Provide oxygen, place in sitting position. May need artificial ventilation.
Hydrogen cyanide: Colorless gas or liquid with a characteristic odor	Highly irritating; symptoms may be immediate or delayed	Headache, confusion, drowsiness, dyspnea, loss of consciousness, nausea, skin and eye redness and pain, burning sensation Enters the body through inhalation, ingestion, eye and skin absorption Easily absorbed as a vapor or through the skin or eyes	May injure CNS, respiratory, and circulatory systems Exposure may cause death	**Skin:** Flush skin with plenty of water or take a shower. Wear gloves when administering first aid. **Eyes:** Immediately flush eyes with water for 10–15 minutes, then seek eye examination. **Ingestion:** Rinse mouth immediately. Do *not* induce vomiting. **Inhalation:** Provide oxygen, place in sitting position. May need artificial ventilation. Avoid mouth-to-mouth resuscitation.

ACLS, advanced cardiac life support; CNS, central nervous system

Communicable Diseases, Colds Versus Flu, and Sexually Transmitted Diseases

COMMUNICABLE DISEASES			
Disease	Mode of Transmission	Incubation Period	Contagious Period
AIDS/HIV	Blood, breast milk, body tissues, fluids exchanged during sexual contact Other body fluids: saliva, urine, tears, bronchial secretions (especially if blood is present)	Variable incubation rates Virus exposure to seroconversion (HIV+): about 1-3 months HIV+ to AIDS: from <1 to 10 years	Although unknown, it is believed to begin just after onset of HIV infection and extend throughout life
Botulism	Contaminated food products	Within 12-36 hours of consumption, up to several days	Not contagious from secondary person-to-person contact
Bronchiolitis	Respiratory	4-6 days	Onset of cough until 7 days
Chancroid	Direct sexual contact with open or draining lesions	3-5 days, up to 14 days	Until treated with antibiotic and lesions healed–usually about 1-2 weeks
Chickenpox (varicella)	Direct person-to-person contact, respiratory droplets	Commonly 14-16 days	1-5 days before the onset of the rash until all sores have crusted over–usually 10-21 days

(*continued*)

Disease	Mode of Transmission	Incubation Period	Contagious Period
Chlamydia infection	Sexual intercourse	Approximately a minimum of 7–14 days	Unknown
Clostridioides difficile infection A bacterial infection that occurs in people with weakened immune systems who have taken antibiotics	Direct contact and indirect contact	~7 days	Contagious when symptomatic, and possibly during latent periods
"Cold," cough, croup	Respiratory	2–5 days	Onset of runny nose and/or cough until fever is gone
Conjunctivitis, viral	Direct or indirect contact	1–12 days	4–14 days after onset of symptoms (minimally contagious)
Conjunctivitis, bacterial	Respiratory, direct contact with eye drainage	24–72 hours	Until treated with antibiotics
Ebola virus infection	Direct or indirect contact, body fluids	2–21 days	From the time symptoms appear and continuing for ~3 months after the illness; a body remains contagious after death
Fifth disease	Respiratory	Variable; 4–20 days	7 days before rash develops, probably not communicable after rash starts
Giardia infection	Fecal contamination of food or water	3–25 days	Entire period of infection, often months
Gonorrhea	Sexual contact	2–7 days	Continues until treatment begins

(continued)

Disease	Mode of Transmission	Incubation Period	Contagious Period
Hand-foot-and-mouth disease (coxsackie virus infection)	Direct contact with nasal or throat secretions, fecal material droplets	3–6 days	Onset of mouth ulcers until fever gone–perhaps as long as several weeks with fecal contamination
Hepatitis A	Fecal-oral route, food contamination	15–50 days	During last half of incubation period until after first week of jaundice
Hepatitis B	Blood, saliva, semen, vaginal fluid	45–180 days	Infective many weeks before onset of first symptom, until completion of acute clinical course of infection
Hepatitis C	Blood and plasma, percutaneous exposure	2 weeks to 6 months	From 1+ weeks before onset of symptoms; may persist indefinitely
Herpes simplex, type 1	Saliva	2–12 days	From onset of sores to 7 weeks after recovery from stomatitis
Herpes simplex, type 2	Sexual contact (oral or genital)	2–12 days	7–12 days
Herpes zoster/shingles (varicella zoster virus infection)	Soiled dressings or articles	Can be 2–3 weeks	1–5 days before the onset of the rash until all sores have crusted over–usually 10–21 days
Impetigo			
Impetigo, Staphylococcus	Hand to skin contact	4–10 days	Until draining lesions heal
Impetigo, *Streptococcus*	Respiratory droplet, direct contact	1–3 days	Untreated: weeks or months Treated: 24 hours on antibiotics
Influenza	Airborne, direct contact	1–3 days	Children: 7 days Adults: 3–5 days
Kawasaki disease	Unknown, seasonal variation	Unknown	Unknown
Legionnaire pneumonia	Airborne	2–16 days	Spreads through mist or moisture in the air

(continued)

Disease	Mode of Transmission	Incubation Period	Contagious Period
Lice, head/body	Direct contact, indirect contact with objects	7–13 days	Continuous if alive, until first treatment; live off host for 7–21 days
Lice, pubic (crabs)	Sexual contact	Egg-to-egg cycle lasts 3 weeks	Live off host for 2 days
Lyme disease	Tickborne	3–32 days	Person to person: none
Measles (rubeola)	Airborne, direct contact with nasal secretions	7–18 days	Before the onset of symptoms to 4 days after the appearance of the rash
Meningitis, bacterial: *Meningococcus*	Direct contact, respiratory, droplet from nose and mouth	2–10 days	Usually after 24 hours on antibiotic therapy
Meningitis, bacterial: *Haemophilus*	Droplet from nose and mouth	2–4 days	Noncommunicable within 24–48 hours on antibiotic therapy
Meningitis, viral	Varies with specific infectious agent		Variable; often 3–7 days
Mononucleosis	Saliva	4–6 weeks	Prolonged, possibly a year
Norovirus infection	Direct or indirect contact (fecal/oral), airborne	12–48 hours	Onset of symptoms up to 2 weeks after recovery
Pertussis	Direct contact, airborne droplet	6–20 days	Gradually decreases over 3 weeks
Pinworms	Direct transfer (anus to mouth), indirect contact (infested bed, etc.)	2–6 weeks	As long as females are alive, eggs survive for about 2 weeks
Rabies	Saliva, direct contact (bite, scratch), indirect contact	3–8 weeks	3–7 days before the onset of symptoms
Ringworm: tinea capitis (scalp)	Direct skin to skin, indirect contact (cloth seats, combs, etc.)	10–14 days	Viable fungus may persist on contaminated articles for long periods of time

Disease	Mode of Transmission	Incubation Period	Contagious Period
Ringworm: tinea corporis (body)	Direct or indirect contact with infected people, articles, floors, benches, animals, shower stalls	4–10 days	While lesions are present and as long as viable fungus remains on articles
Rocky Mountain spotted fever	Tickborne	3–14 days	Noncommunicable person to person; tick remains infective for life, as long as 18 months
Roseola	Unknown, possibly saliva	10–15 days	Onset of fever until rash is gone
Rotavirus infection	Fecal–oral route, possible respiratory	24–72 hours	Average 4–6 days
Rubella	Direct contact with nasal secretions, droplet	14–23 days	1 week before to at least 4 days after onset of rash
Salmonella infection	Ingestion of contaminated food	6–72 hours	Throughout the course of infection
Scabies	Direct skin-to-skin contact	2–6 weeks	Until mites and eggs are destroyed
Scarlet fever	Large respiratory droplet, direct contact	1–3 days	Untreated: 10–21 days Treated: 24 hours of antibiotic therapy
Shigella infection	Fecal–oral route, ingestion of contaminated food	12–96 hours	During acute infection until infectious agent no longer in feces (about 4 weeks)
Sore throat, streptococcal	Large respiratory droplet, direct contact	1–3 days	Untreated: 10–21 days Treated: after 24 hours of antibiotic therapy
Sore throat, viral	Direct contact, inhalation of airborne droplet	1–5 days	Onset of sore throat until fever gone

(*continued*)

Disease	Mode of Transmission	Incubation Period	Contagious Period
Syphilis	Direct contact with moist lesions and body fluids	10 days to 3 months	Untreated: variable and indefinite Treated: after 24–48 hours of antibiotic therapy
Tetanus	Spores enter open wound	3–21 days	Noncommunicable from person to person
Trichomoniasis	Sexual contact through vaginal or urethral secretions	4–24 days	Untreated: may be symptom-free carrier for years
Tuberculosis	Airborne droplet	4–12 weeks	Degree of communicability depends on many factors; treated: within a few weeks; children usually not infectious

"COLD" VS. FLU SYMPTOM COMPARISON

Symptom	"Cold"	Flu
Fever	Rare	Usually high (102°F–104°F); lasts 3–4 days
Headache	Rare	Yes
Body aches and pains	Slight	Often severe
Fatigue	Mild	Lasts 2–3 weeks
Extreme exhaustion	No	Early in illness; lasts a few days
Stuffy or runny nose	Yes	Occasionally
Sneezing	Yes	Occasionally
Sore throat	Yes	Occasionally
Chest discomfort and/or cough	Mild to moderate; hacking cough	Yes; may be severe
Complications	Sinus congestion, ear pain	Bronchitis, pneumonia

SEXUALLY TRANSMITTED DISEASES

Disease	Clinical Presentation	Complications and Long-Term Risks
AIDS/HIV	May remain asymptomatic for many years Developing signs and symptoms include fatigue, fever, poor appetite, unexplained weight loss, generalized lymphadenopathy, persistent diarrhea, night sweats	Disease progression (from HIV to AIDS) is variable from a few months to 12 years. Early intervention is essential in preserving and maintaining optimal health status.
Chancroid	Painful genital ulceration(s) with tender inguinal adenopathy Ulcers may be necrotic or erosive	Chancroid has been associated with increased risk of acquiring HIV infection. Patients should be tested for other infections that cause ulcers (i.e., syphilis).
Chlamydial cervicitis	Yellow mucopurulent cervical exudate May or may not be symptomatic Male sexual partner will likely have nongonococcal urethritis	Untreated, may develop endometritis, salpingitis, ectopic pregnancy, and/or subsequent infertility. High prevalence of coinfection with gonococcal infection. Infection during pregnancy may lead to premature rupture of membranes, pneumonia, or conjunctivitis in the infant.
Enteric infections	Sexually transmissible enteric infections, particularly among homosexual males Abdominal pain, fever, diarrhea, vomiting	Occurs frequently with oral–genital and oral–anal contact. Infections can be life threatening if they become systemic. Organisms may be *Shigella*, hepatitis A virus, *Giardia*.
Epididymitis	May or may not be transmitted sexually Can be asymptomatic Nonsexually transmitted Associated with a urinary tract infection Unilateral testicular pain and swelling	Usually caused by gonorrhea or *Chlamydia* infection. May be caused by *Escherichia coli* after anal intercourse. Must rule out a testicular torsion before making the diagnosis of epididymitis.
Genital warts	Soft, fleshy, painless growth(s) around the anus, penis, vulvovaginal area, cervix, urethra, or perineum	Caused by the human papillomavirus. Must rule out other causes of lesion(s) such as syphilis, etc. Lesions may cause tissue destruction. Cervical warts are associated with neoplasia.

(continued)

Disease	Clinical Presentation	Complications and Long-Term Risks
Gonorrhea	Males may have dysuria, urinary frequency, thin clear or yellow urethral discharge Females may have mucopurulent vaginal discharge, abnormal menses, dysuria, or no symptoms	Untreated, risk of arthritis, dermatitis, bacteremia, meningitis, endocarditis. At risk: Males: epididymitis, infertility, urethral stricture, and sterility Females: PID Newborns: ophthalmia neonatorum, pneumonia
Hepatitis B	Anorexia, malaise, nausea, vomiting, abdominal pain, jaundice, skin rash, arthralgias, arthritis	Chronic hepatitis, cirrhosis, liver cancer, liver failure, death Chronic carrier occurs in 6%–10% of cases. Infants born with hepatitis B are at high risk for developing chronic liver disease.
Herpes genitalis (herpes simplex, type 2)	Clustered vesicles that rupture, leaving painful, shallow genital ulcer(s) that eventually crust Initial outbreak lasts 14–21 days; subsequent outbreaks are less severe and last 8–12 days	Other causes of genital ulcers (syphilis, chancroid, etc.) must be ruled out.
Nongonococcal urethritis	Dysuria, urinary frequency, mucoid to purulent urethral discharge Some men may be asymptomatic Female sexual partners may have cervicitis or PID	Can be caused by *Chlamydia*, *Mycoplasma*, *Trichomonas*, or herpes simplex virus; can cause urethral strictures, prostatitis, epididymitis.
PID	Lower abdominal pain, fever, cervical motion tenderness, dyspareunia, purulent vaginal discharge, dysuria, increased abdominal pain while walking	Must rule out appendicitis or ectopic pregnancy. Risk for pelvic abscess, future ectopic pregnancy, infertility, pelvic adhesions.
Proctitis	Sexually transmitted gastrointestinal illnesses Proctitis occurs with anal intercourse, resulting in inflammation of the rectum with anorectal pain, tenesmus, and rectal discharge	May be caused by *Chlamydia* infection, gonorrhea, herpes simplex, and syphilis. Among patients coinfected with HIV, herpes proctitis may be severe.

(continued)

Disease	Clinical Presentation	Complications and Long-Term Risks
Proctocolitis	Sexually transmitted gastro-intestinal illnesses Proctocolitis occurs with either anal intercourse or with oral-fecal contact, resulting in symptoms of proctitis as well as diarrhea, abdominal cramps, and inflammation of the colonic mucosa	May be caused by *Campylobacter, Shigella,* or *Chlamydia.* Other opportunistic infections may be involved among immunosuppressed HIV patients.
Pubic lice	Slight discomfort to intense itching May have pruritic, erythematous macules, papules, or secondary excoriation in the genital area If lice are found on the eyelashes, they are usually pubic lice	Sexual partners within the last month should be treated. May develop lymphadenitis or a secondary bacterial infection of the skin or hair follicle.
Scabies	The mite burrows under the skin of the fingers, penis, and wrists Scabies among adults may be sexually transmitted, while usually *not* sexually transmitted among children Itching (worse at night), papular eruptions, and excoriation of the skin	Sexual partners, household members, and close contacts within the past month should be examined and treated. May develop a secondary infection, often with nephritogenic streptococci.
Syphilis		
Primary syphilis	Painless, indurated ulcer (chancre) at site of infection ~10 days to 3 months after exposure	All genital ulcers should be suspected to be syphilitic. Patients should be tested for HIV and retested in 3 months. At-risk sex partners are those within the past 3 months plus duration of symptoms for primary syphilis, and 6 months plus duration of symptoms for secondary syphilis.
Secondary syphilis	Rash, mucocutaneous lesions, lymphadenopathy, condylomata lata Symptoms occur 4–6 weeks after exposure and resolve spontaneously within weeks to 12 months	

(continued)

Disease	Clinical Presentation	Complications and Long-Term Risks
Latent syphilis	Seroreactive yet asymptomatic Can be clinically latent for a period of weeks to years Latency sometimes lasts a lifetime	Should be clinically evaluated for tertiary disease (aortitis, neurosyphilis, etc.). At-risk sex partners are those within the past year for early latent syphilis.
Tertiary/late syphilis	May have cardiac, neurologic, ophthalmic, auditory, or gummatous lesions	Occurs 3–10 years after initial infection.
Neurosyphilis	May see a variety of neurologic signs and symptoms, including ataxia, bladder problems, confusion, meningitis, uveitis May be asymptomatic	Diagnosis made based on a variety of tests including reactive serologic test results, CSF protein or cell count abnormalities, positive VDRL on CSF.
Congenital syphilis	Needs to be ruled out for infants born to mothers with untreated syphilis, mothers who received incomplete treatment, or insufficient follow-up of reported treated syphilis Serologic tests for mother and infant can be negative at delivery if mother was infected late in pregnancy	Syphilis frequently causes abortion, stillbirth, and complications of prematurity of infant. Treated infants must be followed very closely and retested every 2–3 months. Most infants are nonreactive by 6 months. Infants with positive CSF should be retested every 6 months and be re-treated if still abnormal at 2 years.
Trichomoniasis (vaginitis)	Profuse, thin, foamy, greenish yellow discharge with foul odor May be asymptomatic Male partners may have urethritis	Trichomoniasis often coexists with gonorrhea. Perform a complete STD assessment if trichomoniasis is diagnosed.

CSF, cerebrospinal fluid; PID, pelvic inflammatory disease; STD, sexually transmitted disease; VDRL, venereal disease research laboratory.

Source: Reproduced with permission from Grossman, V. (2003). *Quick reference to triage* (2nd ed.). Philadelphia, PA: Lippincott Williams & Wilkins.

ACC/AHA/AAPA/ABC/ACPM/AGS/APhA/ASH/ASPC/NMA/PCNA Guideline for the Prevention, Detection, Evaluation, and Management of High Blood Pressure in Adults. (2017). doi:10.1016/j.jacc.2017.11.006. Retrieved from https://doi.org/10.1016/elsevier_cm_policy

Agency for Healthcare Research and Quality. (2014). *Modified Early Warning Score (MEWS)*. Retrieved from https://innovations.ahrq.gov/qualitytools/modified-early-warning-system-mews

American College of Cardiology. (2017). *New ACC/AHA high blood pressure guidelines lower definition of hypertension*. Retrieved from https://www.acc.org/latest-in-cardiology/articles/2017/11/08/11/47/mon-5pm-bp-guideline-aha-2017

American Stroke Association. (n.d.). *Stroke symptoms*. Retrieved from https://www.strokeassociation.org/en/about-stroke/stroke-symptoms

Borchers, A. (Ed.). (2015). *Handbook of signs & symptoms* (5th ed.). Philadelphia, PA: Wolters Kluwer.

Briggs, J. K. (2016). *Telephone triage protocols for nurses* (5th ed.). Philadelphia, PA: Wolters Kluwer.

Briggs, J. K. (2019). *Triage protocols for aging adults*. Philadelphia, PA: Wolters Kluwer.

Briggs, J. K., & Meadows-Oliver, M. (2018). *Telephone triage protocols for pediatrics*. Philadelphia, PA: Wolters Kluwer.

Cafasso, J. (2018). *Anticholinergics*. Retrieved from https://www.healthline.com/health/anticholinergics

Centers for Disease Control and Prevention. (n.d.). *Carbon monoxide poisoning: Frequently asked questions*. Retrieved from https://www.cdc.gov/co/faqs.htm

Centers for Disease Control and Prevention. (n.d.). Clostridioides difficile *infection*. Retrieved from https://www.cdc.gov/hai/organisms/cdiff/cdiff_infect.html

Centers for Disease Control and Prevention. (n.d.). *Norovirus*. Retrieved from https://www.cdc.gov/norovirus/index.html

Christ, M., Grossmann, F., Winter, D., Bingisser, R., & Platz, E. (2010). Modern triage in the emergency department. *Deutsches Arzteblatt International, 107*(50), 892–898. doi:10.3238/arztebl.2010.0892

Crist, C. (2019). Public spaces should stock bleeding-control kits for mass casualties, experts say. *Medscape*. Retrieved from https://www.medscape.com/viewarticle/907573

Department of Homeland Security. (2019). *Preventing terrorism*. Retrieved from https://www.dhs.gov/topic/preventing-terrorism

Domino, F. J., Balder, R. A., Grimes, J., & Grimes, A. (Eds.). (2014). *The 5-minute clinical consult standard 2015* (23rd ed.). Philadelphia, PA: Wolters Kluwer.

FitzGerald, G., Jelinek, G., Scott, D., & Gerdtz, M. (2010). Emergency department triage revisited. *Emergency Medicine Journal, 27*(2), 86–92. doi:10.1136/emj.2009.077081

Glatter, R., & Ho, A. F. (2018). Emergency 'MacGyver' tips for physicians. *Medscape*. Retrieved from https://www.medscape.com/viewarticle/905376

Glatter, R. D., Antevy, P. M., & Sakran, J. V. (2019). 'Stop the Bleed' kits—Preparing everyone for mass casualties. *Medscape*. Retrieved from https://www.medscape.com/viewarticle/907187

Goodwin Veenema, T. (2018). *Disaster nursing and emergency preparedness* (4th ed.). New York, NY: Springer Publishing Company.

Gresham, C. (2018). Benzodiazepine toxicity. In G. Z. Shlamovitz (Ed.), *Medscape*. Retrieved from https://emedicine.medscape.com/article/813255-overview

Hibberd, O., Nuttall, D., Watson, R. E., Watkins, W. J., Kemp, A. M., & Maguire, S. (2017). Childhood bruising distribution observed from eight mechanisms of unintentional injury. *Archives of Disease in Childhood, 102*, 1103–1109. doi:10.1136/archdischild-2017-312847

Hilton, M. T. (2017). How clinicians can prepare for active shooter incidents. *Medscape*. Retrieved from https://www.medscape.com/viewarticle/883992

Kolecki, P. (2018). Sympathomimetic toxicity. In A. Tarabar (Ed.), *Medscape*. Retrieved from https://emedicine.medscape.com/article/818583-overview

Long, V. E., & McMullen, P. C. (Eds.). (2019). *Telephone triage for obstetrics & gynecology* (3rd ed.). Philadelphia, PA: Wolters Kluwer Health.

Mahavar, S., Chaturvedi, A., Singh, A., Kumar, R., Dariya, S., & Sharma, R. (2018). Toluene poisoning presenting as bilateral basal ganglia haemorrhage. *Journal of the Association of Physicians of India, 66*, 93–94. Retrieved from http://www.japi.org/september_2018/19_CR_Toluene_Poisoning_Presenting_as_Bilateral.pdf

Maleki, M., Fallah, R., Riahi, L., Delavari, S., & Rezaei, S. (2015). Effectiveness of five-level emergency severity index triage system compared with three-level spot check: An Iranian experience. *Archives of Trauma Research, 4*(4), e29214. doi:10.5812/atr.29214

McNamara, C., Mironova, I., Lehman, E., & Olympia, R. (2017). Predictors of intrathoracic injury after blunt torso trauma in children presenting to an emergency department as trauma activations. *Journal of Emergency Medicine, 52*(6), 793–800. doi:10.1016/j.jemermed.2016.11.031

Poison Control Center. (n.d.). Retrieved from https://www.webpoisoncontrol.org

Porretto-Loehrke, A., Schuh, C., & Szekeres, M. (2016). Clinical manual assessment of the wrist. *Journal of Hand Therapy, 29*(2), 123–135. doi:10.1016/j.jht.2016.02.008

Psychemedics. (n.d.). *Amphetamine*. Retrieved from https://www.psychemedics.com/amphetamine

Robertson-Steel, I. (2006). Evolution of triage systems. *Emergency Medicine Journal, 23*, 154–155. doi:10.1136/emj.2005.030270

Schaider, J., Hayden, S. R., Wolfe, R., Barkin, R. M., & Rosen, P. (Eds.). (2007). *Rosen & Barkin's 5-minute emergency medicine consult* (3rd ed.). Philadelphia, PA: Lippincott Williams & Wilkins.

Tam, H. L., Chung, S. F., & Lou, C. K. (2018). A review of triage accuracy and future direction. *BMC Emergency Medicine, 18*(1), 58. doi:10.1186/s12873-018-0215-0

The Interagency Board. (2017). *Training trigger: Tourniquet use under medical protocols*. Retrieved from www.interagencyboard.org

Tscheschlog, B. A., & Jauch, A. (Eds.). (2015). *Emergency nursing made incredibly easy!* (2nd ed.). Philadelphia, PA: Wolters Kluwer.

U.S. Department of Health and Human Services. (2019). *Anticholinergic agents (anticholinergic toxidrome).* Chemical Hazards of Emergency Medical Management. Retrieved from https://chemm.nlm.nih.gov/anticholinergic.htm

Visser, L., & Montejano, A. (2018). *Rapid access guide for triage and emergency nurses.* New York, NY: Springer Publishing Company.

Visser, L., & Montejano, A. (Eds.). (2019). *Fast facts for the triage nurse* (2nd ed.). New York, NY: Springer Publishing Company.

Whelton, P. K., Carey, R. M., Aronow, W. S., Casey, D. E., Jr., Collins, K. J., Dennison Himmelfarb, C., . . . Wright, J. T., Jr. (2018). 2017 ACC/AHA/AAPA/ABC/ACPM/AGS/APhA/ASH/ASPC/NMA/PCNA guideline for the prevention, detection, evaluation, and management of high blood pressure in adults. *Journal of the American College of Cardiology, 71*(19), e127–e248. doi:10.1016/j.jacc.2017.11.006

Williams, M., & Sizemore, D. C. (2018). *Biologic, chemical, and radiation terrorism review.* Treasure Island, FL: StatPearls Publishing. Retrieved from https://www.ncbi.nlm.nih.gov/books/NBK493217

World Health Organization. (2017). *Emergency preparedness, response: Frequently asked questions on Ebola virus disease.* Retrieved from https://www.who.int/csr/disease/ebola/faq-ebola/en

World Health Organization. (2018). *Female genital mutilation.* Retrieved from https://www.who.int/news-room/fact-sheets/detail/female-genital-mutilation

INDEX

Printed in the United States
by Baker & Taylor Publisher Services